GET YOUR BEACH BODY IN 4 WEEKS

WORKOUT AND NUTRITION TIPS TO BUILD YOUR SUMMER BODY IN A MONTH

THOMAS FREY

© Copyright 2021 by Thomas Frey

All rights reserved.

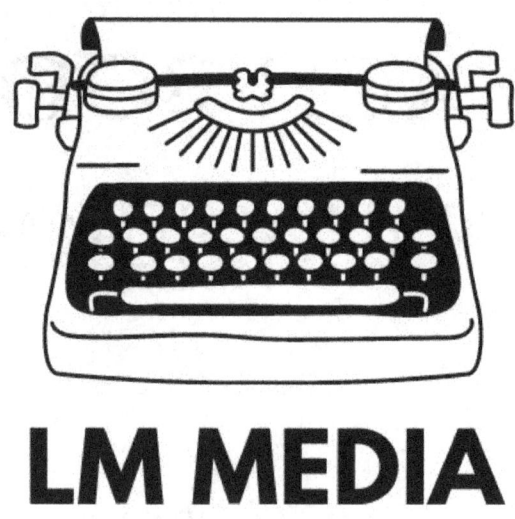

ISBN: 978-1-80232-492-1

The content of this book may not be reproduced, duplicated or transmitted without direct written permission from the author or the publisher.

Under no circumstances will any blame or legal responsibility be held against the publisher, or author, for any damages, reparation, or monetary loss due to the information contained within this book, either directly or indirectly.

Legal Notice:

This book is copyright protected. It is only for personal use. You cannot amend, distribute, sell, use, quote or paraphrase any part, or the content within this book, without the author or publisher's consent.

All pictures contained in this book come from the author's personal archive or copyright-free stock websites (Pixabay, Pexel, Freepix, Unsplash, StockSnap, etc.).

Disclaimer Notice:

Please note the information contained within this document is for educational and entertainment purposes only. All effort has been executed to present accurate, up-to-date, reliable, complete information. No warranties of any kind are declared or implied. Readers acknowledge that the author is not engaged in the rendering of legal, financial, medical or professional advice. The content within this book has been derived from various sources. Please consult a licensed professional before attempting any techniques outlined in this book.

By reading this document, the reader agrees that under no circumstances is the author responsible for any losses, direct or indirect, that are incurred as a result of the use of the information contained within this document, including, but not limited to, errors, omissions, or inaccuracies.

The trademarks used are without any consent, and the publication of the trademark is without permission or backing by the trademark owner. All trademarks and brands within this book are for clarifying purposes only and are owned by the owners themselves, not affiliated with this document.

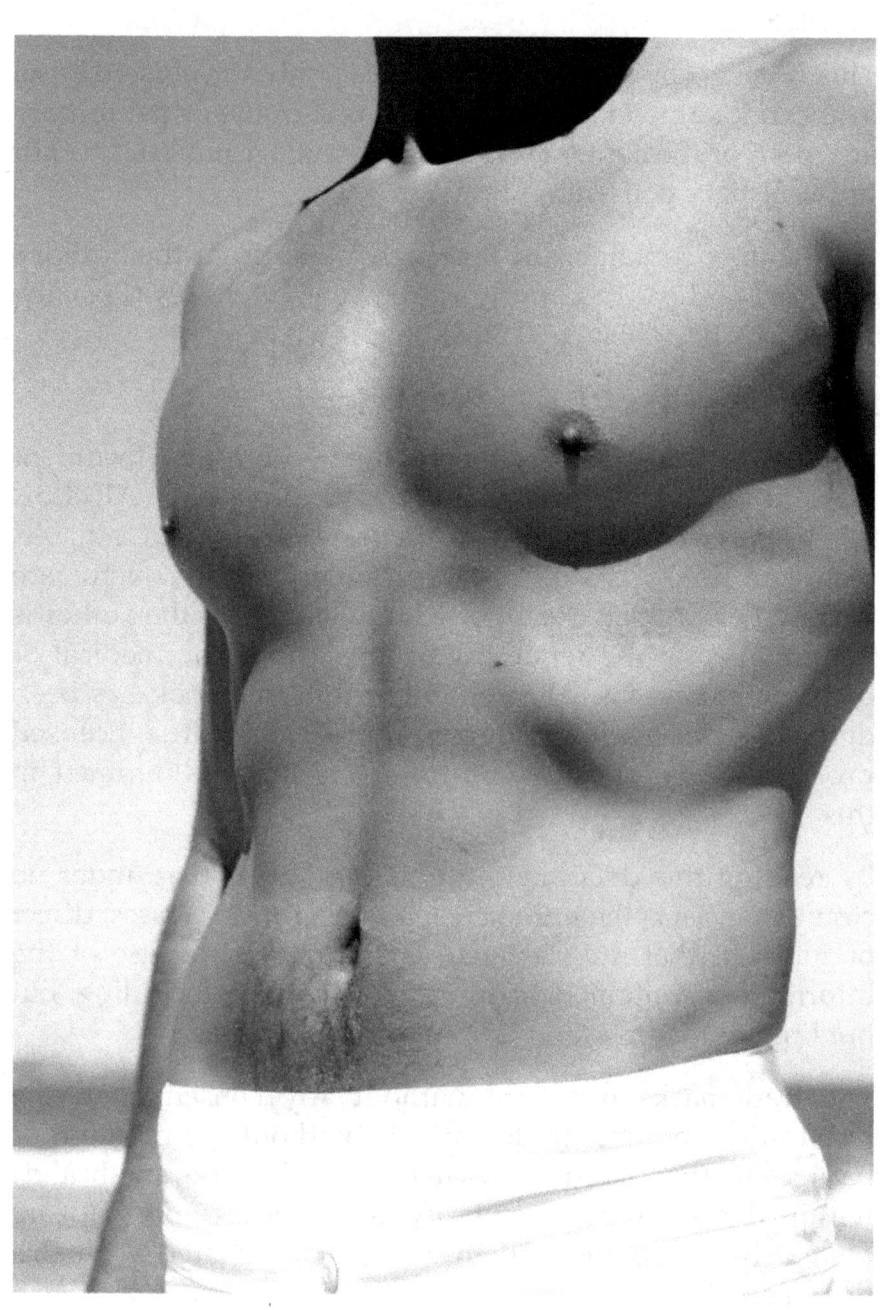

TABLE OF CONTENTS

INTRODUCTION 1

4 WEEKS TO... A BEACH BODY 3

   Reasons Summer is the Best Time to Get Fit 3

   4 Weeks to go 6

   3 Weeks to go 7

   2 Weeks to go 8

   1 Week to go 10

THE HEALTHY MINDSET TO GET THAT SUMMER BODY 12

EXERCISE IS THE KEY TO A PERFECT SHAPED BODY 17

   Reasons to get and stay in shape 18

MENTAL HEALTH BENEFITS OF WORKOUT 24

   What are the mental health benefits of exercise? 25

   Reaping the mental health benefits of exercise is easier ...27

   than you think 27

   Overcoming obstacles to exercise 29

   Beginning with practice when you have an emotional 30

   wellness issue 30

5 EXTRA MENTAL BENEFITS OF EXERCISE 33

   The Psychological Benefits of Exercise 33

PROVEN BENEFITS OF PHYSICAL ACTIVITY 36

   How much physical activity should we do? 40

   Top Benefits of Strength Training 43

THE BEACH BODY WORKOUT 47

   The Warm-up 47

   The Schedule 49

   The Moves 50

   The Training Plan Explained 54

   Block 1 - Week 1 57

   Square 1 - Week 2 63

   Square 2: Week 1 66

   Saturday Workout: Delts And Abs 70

   Square 2 - Week 2 71

THE BEST BEACH BODY DIET 79

   It all comes down to calories 79

   Take note of the macros 80

   Consume just healthy foods 82

   Training's Role 83

   What's the Best Food to Eat After a Workout? 84

   6 Superfoods to Get a Beach Body 87

   Tips to Get Beach Body Quickly 89

   Top 6 Foods to Avoid for a Beach Body 95

How to prevent bloating after a meal.................................99
OBSTACLE IN OUR PATH..104
6 Common Issues When Getting Fit....................................104
Negative Mind Patterns When Getting Fit........................107
MOTIVATIONAL QUOTES TO INSPIRE YOU TOWARD YOUR GOAL..115

INTRODUCTION

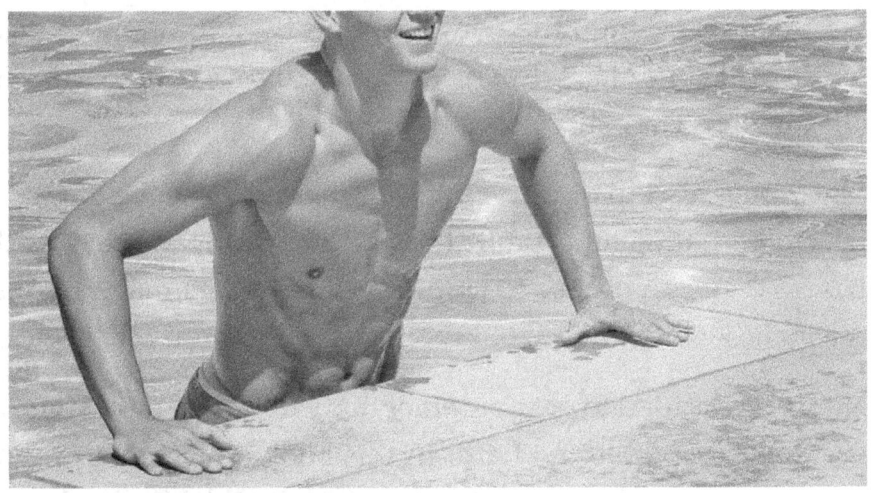

One of the most important aspects of getting in shape for summer is to begin before it arrives! It's just around the corner, so don't put it off until August 1st to decide it's time to get in shape.

To really see the best results, give yourself at least four weeks – when I really want to get in phenomenal shape, I give my body nine weeks to see optimum results. So, if you have a month, let's get started right away!

With the arrival of warmer weather, there is plenty we can do to get physically fit in time for summer. Remember that a happy person exists in a perfect body. It's happening once more. The same thing happened the previous year and the year before that. Summer!

One minute it's Christmas, with all of the calorific indulgence that entails, and the next thing we know, Valentine's Day has wrapped its loving little wings around us, adding more inches to our waistline. That doesn't even take into account Easter and anything else in between.

Many people's top priority until summer is to lose weight. We've been hibernating and comfort-eating all winter, and the weather has given us an excuse to skip the gym. Others may not notice the inches we've added, but we do.

Now you decided to get a summer body to show off on your next vacation, prepare to go hard. In this book, you find a program designed to assist you with all the necessities, including benefits analysis, workout advice, healthy diet tips, and motivational quotes.

Every week in the program will bring more challenging exercises, yet you'll adore the final result: The perfect beach body!

4 WEEKS TO... A BEACH BODY

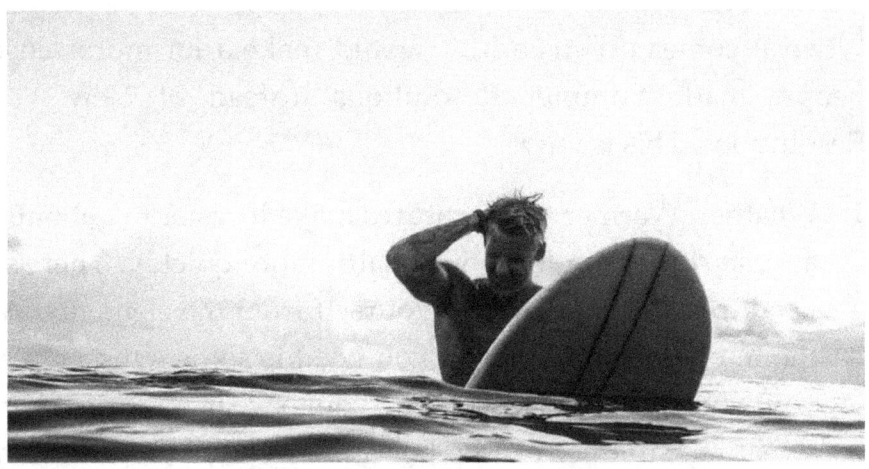

Why Summer is the Best Time to Get Fit

The most commonly associated time of year with getting well is January 1st. People adore a healthy New Year's resolution, regardless of how likely–or, more often, unlikely–they are to keep it. There's something about the start of the year that makes people think, "New year, new me!"

Setting goals is still a good idea, regardless of the season. The season, on the other hand, makes January 1st difficult. The duration immediately following the holidays is tough. Not only have you possibly snacked excessively and dropped out of your daily routine as a result of holiday celebrations and gift shopping, but the days are shorter, making it impossible to stay motivated all day. Then there's the weather. It's cold outside in many parts of the country–very cold, as in, there's no way in hell I want to leave my house and do something cold. Feeling this way may make a trip to the gym seem implausible, adding to the difficulty of establishing new healthy habits.

When it comes down to it, it would make a lot more sense if people made Summer Resolutions instead of New Year's Resolutions. This is why:

1. Weather: Warmer temperatures make it easier to get outside and start focusing on your health more quickly. There's no need to cover up to shield yourself from the elements. With the temperature rising, all you need is some sunscreen and your everyday clothes to get your sweat on. Speaking of sweating, summer can be hot and sweaty, but you can still fight the heat by swimming laps or choosing a shaded bike path. Working out in the winter is not the same. When it's cold outside, it's cold outside.
2. Produce: Eating healthy is important for achieving the body of your dreams, and summer is the ideal time of year for new and local foods. Farmers' markets are brimming with a rainbow of vegetables and fruits that are sure to please even the pickiest of eaters. Warmer weather causes you to eat less, while cold weather causes you to eat hearty foods that fill you up but also weigh you down.
3. Motivation: Let's face it: it's easy to conceal excess body fat in the winter when you're covered under layers of thermal and fleece. However, in the summer, lightweight clothes, sleeveless tops, shorts, and, of course, swimsuits expose more of your body. Although you should love your body regardless of its appearance, summer clothing may provide

the encouragement you need to get on a healthier path that will lead to a more confident you.
4. Outdoor Activities: While skiing, snowboarding, and ice skating are available in the winter if you live in an area that has them, the summer sweat opportunities seem limitless. Hiking, stand-up paddle boarding, surfing, diving, riding, rock climbing, skateboarding, canoeing, kayaking, sailing...need we say more? We will definitely do so. Summer is jam-packed with opportunities–take advantage of one!
5. Day Length: While winter can make you want to hibernate, summer's longer days and more hours of sunlight will make getting out of bed and working out in the morning that much easier. Evening workout is a healthy option if you need to get rid of the tension of the day.
6. Group Activities: Gatherings with friends in the winter are often focused on food and drink. Summer gatherings, on the other hand, feel more involved. A backyard barbecue can quickly devolve into a bocce tournament. In addition to swimming and body surfing, a day at the beach can include Frisbee throwing and a sand volleyball match.

Don't worry if you failed to keep your New Year's resolution; you're not alone. Now that summer is close, revisit your goals from the beginning of the year and see if you can't make them last this summer. Give it a shot, and you might be shocked at how simple they feel when the sun is shining. And, as an added bonus, forming the behaviors now means you won't need to make any winter resolutions because you'll already be a better version of yourself!

Get in shape for the season!

The vacation has been reserved. Follow this blueprint to looking good by the sea for muscle and weight-loss gains as assured as your shady passport picture...

4 Weeks to go

<u>Exercise</u>

Switch your metabolic dial to 'incinerate' to distract those on the sand from the fact that your skin is causing glare problems for the lifeguard. Your month-long belly offensive will get off to the best possible start with high-intensity interval training. According to a report published in the Journal of Applied Nutrition Physiology and Metabolism, it raises your body's potential for fat burning by 60%, increasing the efficacy of all the exercise you'll do in the coming weeks.

Mike Travis, a trainer of trainers who runs gyms all over London, recommends riding a bike or cross-trainer as hard and quick as you can for 30 seconds. Then pause for 2 minutes before repeating – that's two intervals. Add an additional 2 every other exercise to keep those fat layers at bay and muscle definition at its peak. "Supplement this with 30-60 minutes of moderate aerobic exercise of your choosing three days this week, from the treadmill to swimming or tennis," Mike continues. You've only lost 1.6 pounds.

<u>Food and nutrition</u>

Forget about cliff-edge diets where calories are drastically reduced. Instead, for the next four weeks, reduce the calorie consumption by one-sixth. Cut out inter-meal snacks and evening carbohydrates for five days this week. "This calorie restriction prevents the metabolic slowdown caused by dramatic dieting," says nutritionist Anita Bolton. "In response to a smaller deficit, the body will oxidize more fat."

This week, boost your zinc levels – according to studies published in the American Journal of Clinical Nutrition, this improves your physical health. Twice a week, eat a lean 200g steak sandwich, which keeps you zinc-rich and protein-rich. You may need it.

Get any sun before the holiday. According to a study conducted by the University of Minnesota, people with higher vitamin D levels (as a result of sun exposure) lost more weight than those with lower levels. If the sun is still barred from entering the UK, boil two eggs for breakfast – you'll get nearly half of your vitamin D RDA from your troops.

3 Weeks to go

<u>Exercise</u>

With your metabolism revved up, it's time to ramp up your conventional weight-training regimen. "Explosive weight training produces faster results because it produces more muscle tension than other forms of resistance training," explains Travis. "Aim to complete an exercise's pushing process in 1 second and the recovery phase in 2-3 seconds." According to research from the Federal University of Rio de Janeiro, doing so raises muscle power 3.5 times more than regular exercise.

"The best upper-body movements for explosive training are dumbbell routines including bicep twists, shoulder lifts, and lateral raises." If that fails, try lifting her suitcase of shoes from the top of the wardrobe.

Food and nutrition

Match your work rate in the gym by allowing your muscles to rest for an extended time. Bean recommends increasing your weekly protein intake by one-fifth starting now. "Add the equivalent of a tin of beans, a boiled egg, and a can of tuna somewhere in your regular diet," she advises.

According to studies from the University of Buffalo in the United States, swimming will improve your respiratory endurance by 38%, making your increased weight program easier to manage. Sprint 2 lengths of the pool 6-10 times with a brief rest in between to emerge from the sea looking like Daniel Craig rather than a lost whale.

2 Weeks to go

Exercise

Your out-of-office email is flawless, and you've been practicing with your new snorkel in the tub. You need to put your muscles to the test after startling them into motion last week if you want to turn heads for anything other than your lobster-like complexion. Include a 15-minute kettlebell workout in your daily weight-lifting routine.

Unsurprisingly, a cannonball on a stick produces results quickly. Perform a 15-minute workout consisting of two-arm kettlebell swings, snatches and cleans, squats, and presses. According to British Lifting Federation trainer James Shilton, aim for 16-24kg with 60 seconds between each exercise three days a week. "This routine focuses on all of the main muscle groups." And your weight loss will peak this week with a 2lb loss.

Food and nutrition

With a fortnight to go, cut down on carbs; this is one of the most effective short-term weight-loss techniques. Dutch researchers discovered that consuming one carb-free meal a day for two weeks raises the metabolic rate by 81 calories per day when one meal per day contains zero carbohydrates and 70% protein. 3 lean roast pork slices with steamed green vegetables or a big salad with a 150g can of tuna You'll have less to declare around your midsection when you arrive.

You'll need to be extra-disciplined with your diet from now on, so get some shut-eye. Research at Chicago University discovered that after eight and a half hours of sleep, people consumed 24% fewer snacks. A bedside read that stimulates your nerves will help you sleep faster. According to research from the University of Pittsburgh Medical Center, using your brain causes you to put your head down faster.

1 Week to go

<u>Exercise</u>

You've worked hard, like a marathon runner, and now you can only think of one thing. It's time to take it easy for a while. For the last week, focus on aerobic exercises. According to a study published in the journal Metabolism – Clinical and Experimental, people who jogged at half-pace, took a brief rest, and then ran to exhaustion lost the most weight. Double-tap your treadmill job and vaporize the last of your midriff before sunny beaches call.

<u>Food and nutrition</u>

Do you want to have one last fish dinner before you leave? A 2009 study from the University of Iceland in Reykjavik discovered that a diet that included 150g of cod or salmon three days a week facilitated weight loss as compared to a diet that did not include marine life.

But forget about the chips – the last thing you want to do now is ruined all your hard work by eating foods that hide your hard-won abs. "Exclude the following ingredients from your diet completely," Bolton recommends. "French fries, onion rings, all-you-can-eat nachos, fizzy soda, doughnuts, ice cream, cookies, and alcohol." Also, any meal served through the windshield of your car.

For a final blitz on belly fat, force yourself to take cold showers for a week. According to new findings from the National Institutes of Health, being subjected to cold temperatures increases the amount of energy used by thyroid hormones, which speeds up the metabolism. You'll be shivering the whole journey to the beach.

THE HEALTHY MINDSET TO GET THAT SUMMER BODY

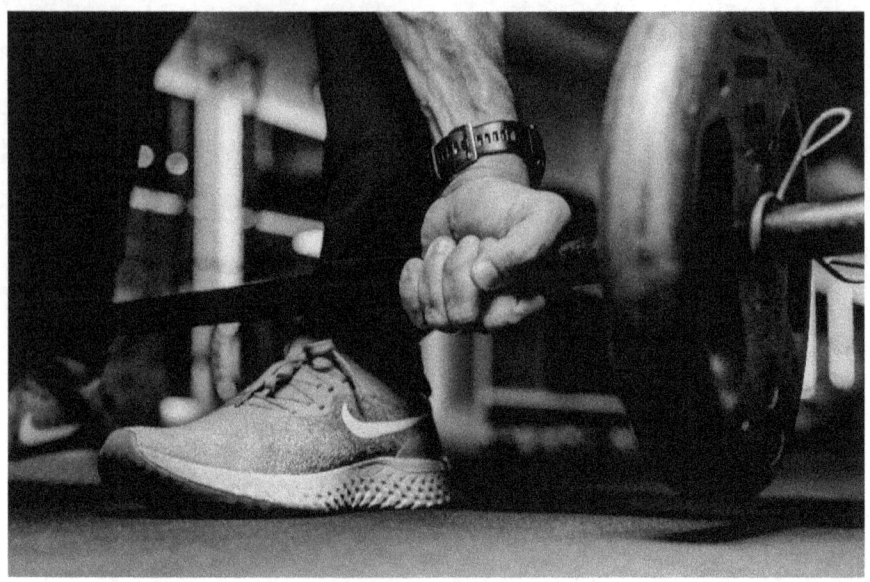

Everyone speaks about getting a summer body, but you'll find that they talk about it year after year, never really doing something, or doing anything and then undoing all of their hard work when summer ends. This is usually because most people do activities that aren't long-term sustainable, such as eating vegetables and exercising twice a day. The truth is that you'll only get a summer body if you're in the right frame of mind. Plus, if you're in the right frame of mind, it won't just be a summer body – it'll be a body you love for the rest of your life. Let's talk about how to get in the right frame of mind so you can actually look the way you've always wanted to:

This Isn't a Short-Term Solution.

To begin, you must recognize that the phrase "summer body" sounds too much like a fast fix, but if you really want to feel good for the near future, it should be a lifestyle change. You've already heard it a million times before, but the best way to get in shape is to make genuine lifestyle changes that you can stick to. If at all possible, avoid putting a time limit on it. If you place too much pressure on yourself, you will become discouraged if your progress slows and end up sabotaging yourself. When you see this as a long-term transition, you will feel less compelled to take drastic action.

The more at ease you are with the situation, the better!!

Stop comparing your journey to that of others.

With social media platforms like Instagram, it's all too tempting to equate your path to someone else's. When you scroll, you see fitness models, and it's easy to start thinking that you're behind or that they look better than you, and this can lead to a negative thought direction, which can lead to a self-sabotage spiral. You must recognize that your path is unique to you and should not be compared to anyone else's. Don't even think about comparing your body to someone else's.

It's fine to be inspired, but you can only help your body become the best version of itself. You would not be able to alter your bone structure or anything else that makes you who you are.

Determine what makes you happy.

When it comes to having a summer body, everyone can tell you different things. There is so much information available that it can be overwhelming, especially for those who are new to the world of health and fitness. To establish a routine that you can adhere to, you must first do something that feels good to you. If you're not having fun, you're not going to stick with it.

Some people want to begin with liposuction, but doing so alone and then returning to your old habits is a bad idea. You must be willing to make the lifestyle change regardless of what else you plan to do. Remember, it's not only about how you look, but also about your attitude and how you feel on the inside. Your mental and physical wellbeing are critical!

Learn to Accept Yourself

In every health and fitness journey, learning to love yourself is important. If you don't love yourself, your efforts would be futile. If you enjoy yourself, you will be more likely to exercise because you want to, rather than because you feel obligated to or as a form of punishment. The same is true when it comes to eating. You'll be more likely to pick balanced, nutritious meals most of the time because you want to have the best possible support for your body. You won't be tempted to eat junk food as much.

Stop Putting Yourself on the Scales

The scale can be especially dangerous to someone who wants to get into the right mindset and get in better shape. Why is this so? Since scales do not show how safe you are – they do not even reflect your weight accurately half of the time. Your weight can fluctuate depending on the scale you stand on, what time of day it is, where you are in your cycle, and other factors. It will fluctuate over the week, so you can't depend on it to provide an accurate representation of your progress.

Instead of measuring yourself, what should you do? Make a mental note of how you feel when you look in the mirror. Examine how your clothes match and how you look.
Examine your satisfaction and stress levels to see if they are changing. Taking measurements is the easiest way to find out if you're getting smaller. Your weight will go up if you've been eating healthy and working out hard, but your measurements can go down, which can confuse many people if they don't realize it! Only don't get too caught up in the numbers. You're heading in the right direction as long as you're consistent.

Reconsider if foods are 'Good' or 'Bad.'

Many people make mistakes by labeling foods as 'healthy' or 'poor.' Food is just food, and the more you believe something is off-limits, the more tempted you would be to eat it. In order to avoid eating food, people normally need to feel free around it. There are no forbidden foods. All should be done in moderation. Make an effort to feel liberated!

EXERCISE IS THE KEY TO A PERFECT SHAPED BODY

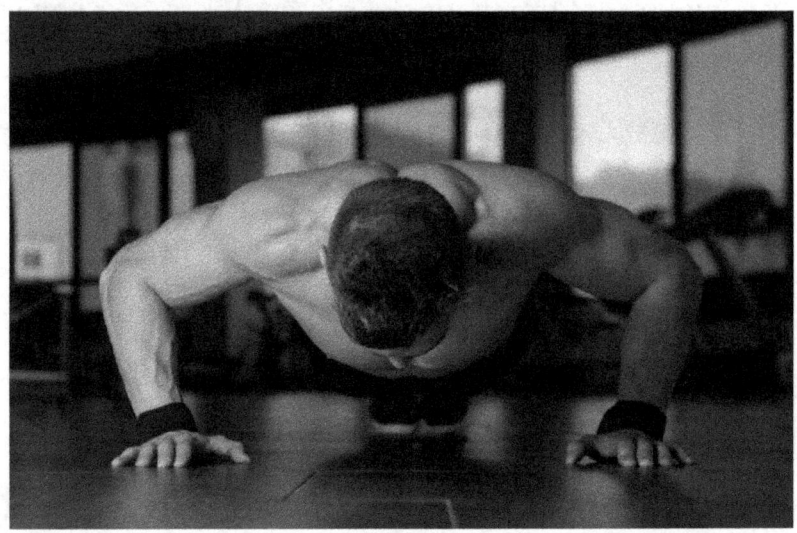

Regular exercise can help assemble slender bulk and give your body definition. This may assist you with accentuating certain highlights or modify your general shape. For instance, you could possibly give your arms more muscle definition with standard training. There are plenty of reasons for being healthy and fit. But most of the time, people hesitate to take any particular exercise. Even they are willing to exercise regularly, but when they find out the schedule and load of exercise, they make their step back. If somebody is making his/her step backward, then it is grunted that he/she will not be benefited and their desire won't come true in the sense of a good physique. Moreover, getting in good shape is not easy at all. It is easy when you are maintaining the formulas and process.

What "getting in good shape" signifies to is you have a pattern of (1) strength, (2) strong perseverance, (3) cardiovascular capacity, and (4) adaptability to lead a more full, better life. Assuming you are frail in one of these 4 zones, you have a hole to fill!

Whenever you're considering skipping activity or you're mulling over getting fit, you can utilize this rundown as an inspirational reference.

Reasons to get and stay in shape

So here are 30 motivations to get or remain in good body shape:

1. Lessens Cholesterol

Standard exercise has been demonstrated to diminish "awful" cholesterol levels (LDL) and increment "great" cholesterol (HDL)

2. Sleep Better

Exercise can help you sleep better. Individuals who exercise will in general nod off faster and stay asleep longer.

3. Develops Self Esteem

Notwithstanding your body appearance, ordinary wellness improves your confidence.

4. Diminishes Blood Pressure

Exercise not just decreases hypertension, it forestalls it.

5. Diminishes Back Pain

By expanding muscle strength, perseverance, and improving adaptability and stance, ordinary exercise assists with forestalling back torment. Studies show that exercise is a compelling treatment for intermittent low back torment.

6. Lessens Risk of Injury

On the off chance that you have a solid, fit body, the odds of injury altogether decline.

7. Forestalls Certain Cancers

A few investigations show that exercise consistently can help decline colon disease hazard by 40% and help diminish the danger of bosom malignancy.

8. Increments Metabolic Rate

Exercise not exclusively will expand the complete number of calories you consume, yet additionally can build your resting metabolic rate, so you consume more calories while still.

9. Expands Range of Motion

An expansion in flexibility can diminish firmness in joints and diminish torment and irritation related to joint inflammation.

10. Increments Functional Strength

From escaping a seat to taking an item off the ground, our bodies can perform everyday exercises better.

11. Builds Insulin Sensitivity

Not exclusively does getting fit as a fiddle help increment insulin affectability (capacity of muscles to take up glucose), yet forestalls type 2 diabetes.

12. Improves Sex Drive

Exercise expands flow, which forestalls erectile brokenness and weakness. Exercise can expand sex hormones like testosterone.

13. Lessens Risk of Heart Disease

Ordinary exercise reinforces the heart and improves contractile capacity

14. Exercise is Fun and Enjoyable

That's right, it's truly obvious. There are such countless approaches to "move" that there will undoubtedly be one you appreciate. Take a stab at making exercise more competitive or social on the off chance that you need additional inspiration. The crucial step obviously is beginning.

15. Exercise Prolongs Life

Individuals who practice consistently watch out for live more.

16. Improves Balance and Coordination

Exercise can improve your strength and furthermore, what is called your "sensation mindfulness." You have a superior vibe of where you are spatially, so you don't thump into things at the supermarket accidentally!

17. Decreases Anxiety and Depression

Exercise is an incredible mindset lift to assist you with overseeing pressure and diminish uneasiness. The upper impact of ordinary actual exercise is similar to the intense antidepressants like Sertraline.

18. Gastrointestinal Tract Benefits

Exercise is advantageous for people experiencing cholelithiasis and blockage. Active work may lessen the danger of diverticulosis, gastrointestinal drain, and incendiary entrails illness.

19. Weight Control

While some exploration shows practice builds hunger, while others show practices smother craving, one thing is without a doubt: routine exercise helps control weight.

20. Improves Fat Utilization

Improves your body's capacity to utilize fat for energy during active work. Our bodies use glycogen and fat to put away energy to help support us.

21. Fortifies Immune System

Pretty much any specialist will reveal to you no pill or healthful enhancement has the force of close to day by day direct movement in bringing down the number of days off individuals take.

22. Reinforces Your Bones

Lifting loads forestalls osteoporosis, which is so significant because a stunning 1 out of 2 ladies will be determined to have osteoporosis.

23. Improves Focus

Exercise improves your cerebrum's capacity to think, recall, picture, prepare and tackle issues because a fitter body will supply a more rich measure of oxygen to your mind.

24. Decreases Aches and Pains

Improves your body's capacity to stand by and be agreeable for significant periods. Keeping your muscles conditioned and solid, and your joints adaptable will keep a throbbing painfulness from diverting you and holding you back from concentrating. If you have office work, practice is a need!

25. Lose the Hidden Fat

However, actually like the fat that prompts stomach rolls and cozy layers, inside fat — called instinctive fat — likewise can be forestalled and killed with standard exercise.

26. Improves Energy Levels

Examination proposes customary exercise can expand energy levels, even among individuals experiencing ongoing ailments related to exhaustion, similar to malignancy and coronary illness. One examination in 2006 showed the normal impact of ordinary exercise was more prominent than the improvement from utilizing energizer prescriptions, like those that treat ADHD and narcolepsy. Disregard some espresso or caffeinated drink, and take a lively walk or exercise!

27. Forestalls Alzheimer's

The most recent exploration shows exercise can keep the cerebrum sharp into mature age and may help forestall Alzheimer's sickness alongside other mental issues that go with maturing.

28. Improves Confidence

While appearance unquestionably isn't all that matters, improving shape can help you look much better and improve your certainty. From the presence of your skin to your general body shape, pretty much every actual trait can improve when you're fit as a fiddle.

29. Arrive at Your Potential

You're not at your best in case you're overweight and rusty. Basically, when you're fit as a fiddle, you're a superior form of YOU, and this actual change can likewise help improve your psychological, passionate, and otherworldly state.

30. Since you can get several hours out of your 168 hour week to get every one of these advantages!

Essentials for getting in good shape are fully defined in these categories. Body and mind connection improvements can be gained through proper exercise. A good physique builds confidence in oneself to make a positive impression on others.

MENTAL HEALTH BENEFITS OF WORKOUT

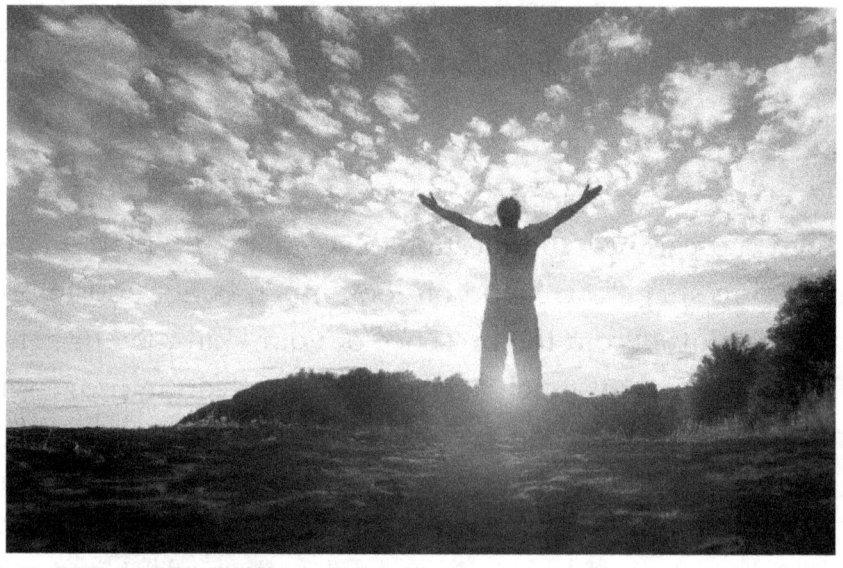

Before getting into how you will get a beach body shape, let's take a tour of the mental and physical essentials and benefits of exercise

You already know that exercise is good for your body. But did you know it can also boost your mood, improve your sleep, and help you deal with depression, anxiety, stress, and more?

What are the mental health benefits of exercise?

Exercise isn't just about the vigorous limits and muscle size. Of course, exercise can improve your actual wellbeing, and your constitution trims your waistline, improve your sexual coexistence, and even add a very long time to your life. Yet, that is not what rouses a great many people to remain dynamic.

Individuals who practice consistently will generally do so because it gives them an immense feeling of prosperity. They feel more vigorous for the duration of the day, rest better around evening time, have more honed recollections, and feel more loose and good about themselves and their lives.

What's more, it's likewise a fantastic medication for some regular psychological wellness challenges.

Regular exercise can affect melancholy, tension, and ADHD. It additionally mitigates pressure, improves memory, assists you with resting better, and supports your general state of mind. What's more, you don't need to be a wellness devotee to receive the rewards. Examination demonstrates that humble measures of activity can have a genuine effect. Regardless of your age or wellness level, you can figure out how to utilize practice as an amazing asset to manage psychological well-being issues, improve your energy and viewpoint, and get more out of life.

<u>Exercise and misery</u>

Studies show that activity can regard gentle to direct sadness as viably as energizer medicine—however, without the results, obviously. As one model, a new report done by the Harvard T.H.

Chan School of Public Health tracked down that running for 15 minutes every day or strolling for an hour lessens the danger of significant misery by 26%. Notwithstanding relieving depression manifestations, research likewise shows that keeping an activity timetable can keep you from backsliding.

Exercise is an amazing misery contender for a few reasons. In particular, it advances a wide range of changes in the cerebrum, including neural development, decreased irritation, and new action designs that advance sensations of quiet and prosperity. It likewise delivers endorphins, incredible synthetics in your mind that invigorate your spirits and cause you to feel better. At last, exercise can likewise fill in as an interruption, permitting you to figure out some tranquil opportunity to break out of the pattern of negative contemplations that feed gloom.

Exercise and nervousness

Exercise is a characteristic and effective anti-nervousness treatment. It calms strain and stress, supports physical and mental energy, and improves prosperity through the arrival of endorphins. Anything that makes you move can help, however, you'll get a greater advantage on the off chance that you focus as opposed to daydreaming.

Attempt to see the vibe of your feet hitting the ground, for instance, or the musicality of your breathing, or the sensation of the breeze on your skin. By adding this care component— truly zeroing in on your body and how it feels as you work out— you'll improve your state of being quicker. However, you may likewise have the option to interfere with the progression of consistent concerns going through your mind.

Exercise and stress

At any point, saw how your body feels when you're under stress? Your muscles might be tense, particularly in your face, neck, and shoulders, leaving you with back or neck torment or difficult migraines. You may feel a snugness in your chest, a beating heartbeat, or muscle cramps. Likewise, you may encounter issues like sleep deprivation, indigestion, stomachache, looseness of the bowels, or incessant pee. The concern and inconvenience of every one of these actual indications can this way prompt considerably more pressure, making an endless loop between your brain and body. Practicing is a viable method to break this cycle. Just as delivering endorphins in the cerebrum, active work assists with loosening up the muscles and diminish strain in the body. Since the body and psyche are so firmly connected, when your body feels much improved along these lines, as well, will your brain.

Reaping the mental health benefits of exercise is easier than you think

Even a little bit of activity is better than nothing

If you don't possess energy for 15 or 30 minutes of activity, or if your body advises you to take a break following 5 or 10 minutes, for instance, that is alright, as well. Start with 5-or 10-minute meetings and gradually increment your time. The more you work out, the more energy you'll have, so in the end, you'll feel prepared for somewhat more. The key is to focus on some moderate actual work—anyway little—on most days. As practicing turns into a propensity, you can gradually add additional minutes or attempt various kinds of exercises. If you keep at it, the advantages of the activity will start to pay off.

<u>You don't need to endure to get results</u>

Exploration shows that moderate degrees of activity are best for a great many people. Moderate methods:

1.   That you inhale somewhat heavier than ordinary, yet are not winded. For instance, you ought to have the option to talk with your strolling accomplice yet not effectively sing a melody.

2.   That your body feels hotter as you move, however not overheated or very damp with sweat.

Can't figure out how to practice during the week? Be an end of the week champion

A new report in the United Kingdom found that individuals who press their activity schedules into a couple of meetings during the end of the week experience nearly as numerous medical advantages as those who work out more frequently. So don't let a bustling timetable at work, home, or school be a pardon to keep away from the movement. Get rolling at whatever point you can make the time—your brain and body will much be obliged!

Overcoming obstacles to exercise

In any event, when you realize that activity will help you feel much improved, venturing out is as yet actually quite difficult. Deterrents to practicing are genuine—especially when you're additionally battling with an emotional wellbeing issue.

Here are some regular obstructions and how you can move beyond them.

Feeling exhausted. When you're worn out, discouraged, or focused, it appears to be that working out will simply exacerbate you. In any case, truly active work is a fantastic energizer. Studies show that ordinary exercise can drastically diminish weariness and increment your energy levels. On the off chance that you are genuinely feeling tired, guarantee yourself a fast, 5-minute walk. Odds are, when you get going, you'll have more energy and have the option to stroll for more.

Feeling overwhelmed. When you're focused or discouraged, the prospect of adding another commitment to your bustling everyday timetable can appear to be overpowering. Working out doesn't appear to be down-toearth. If you have youngsters, discovering childcare while you exercise can likewise be a significant obstacle. Notwithstanding, on the off chance that you start considering actual work a need (a need for your psychological prosperity), you'll before long discover approaches to fit limited quantities of activity into even the busiest timetable.

Feeling hopeless. Even on the off chance that you've never worked out, you can, in any case, discover approaches to serenely get dynamic. Start delayed with simple, low-sway exercises a couple of moments every day, like strolling or moving.

Feeling terrible about yourself. Are you your own most noticeably awful pundit? It's an ideal opportunity to attempt another perspective about your body. Regardless of your weight, age, or wellness level, there are a lot of others in a comparable situation. Request that a companion practice with you. Achieving even the littlest wellness objectives will help you acquire body certainty and improve how you consider yourself.

Feeling pain. If you have an incapacity, extreme weight issue, joint inflammation, or any injury or ailment that restricts your versatility, converse with your doctor about approaches to securely work out. You shouldn't overlook torment, but instead, do what you can when you can. Separation your activity into more limited, more continuous pieces of time if that helps, or have a go at practicing in water to diminish joint or muscle uneasiness.

Beginning with practice when you have an emotional wellness issue

A significant number of us think that it's hard enough to rouse ourselves to practice under the most favorable circumstances. Yet, when you feel discouraged, restless, pushed, or have another emotional wellness issue, it can appear to be doubly troublesome. This is particularly valid for misery and tension, leaving you feeling caught in a predicament circumstance. You realize exercise will cause you to feel much improved; however, wretchedness has denied you of the energy and inspiration you need to work out. Your social anxiety means you can't bear the prospect of being seen at an activity class or going through the recreation center.

Start small. When you're under the haze of tension or gloom and haven't practiced for quite a while, defining luxurious objectives like finishing a long-distance race or turning out for an hour each day will possibly leave you more sorrowful on the off chance that you miss the mark. Better to set attainable objectives and develop from that point.

Timetable exercises when your energy is highest. Perhaps you have most energy first thing before work or school or at noon before the mid-evening quiet hits? Or then again, perhaps you improve practicing for more at the ends of the week. If downturn or uneasiness makes them feel drained and unmotivated the entire day, take a stab at moving to some music or just taking a walk. Indeed, even a short, 15minute walk can help clear your psyche, improve your disposition, and lift your energy level. As you move and begin to feel somewhat better, you'll frequently support your energy enough to practice all the more enthusiastically—by strolling further, breaking into a run, or adding a bicycle ride, for instance.

Zero in on exercises you enjoy. Any movement that makes you move tallies. That could incorporate tossing a Frisbee with a canine or companion, strolling laps of a shopping center window shopping, or cycling to the supermarket. If you've never practiced or don't have the foggiest idea of what you may appreciate, attempt a couple of various things. Exercises like cultivating or handling a home improvement can be incredible approaches to begin moving more when you have a state of mind issue—just as assisting you with getting more dynamic, they can likewise leave you with a feeling of direction and achievement.

Be comfortable. Wear happy with garments and pick a setting that you discover quieting or stimulating. That might be a calm corner of your home, a picturesque way, or your number one city park.

Award yourself. Part of the compensation of finishing an action is how much better you'll feel a while later, yet it generally assists your inspiration with promising yourself an additional treat for working out. Prize yourself with a hot air pocket shower after an exercise, a heavenly smoothie, or with an additional scene of your number one TV show, for instance.

Make practice a social activity. Exercising with a companion or adored one, or even your children, won't just make practicing more fun and agreeable. Yet, it can likewise help propel you to adhere to an exercise schedule. You'll additionally feel better compared to on the off chance that you were practicing alone. Indeed, when you're experiencing a state of mind issue like sadness, friendship can be similarly pretty much as significant as exercise.

5 EXTRA MENTAL BENEFITS OF EXERCISE

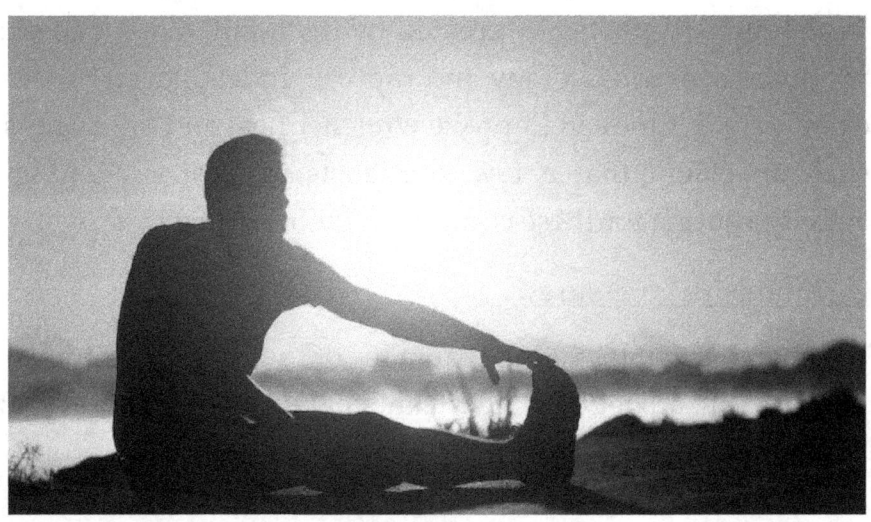

The Psychological Benefits of Exercise

The majority of us know the numerous actual advantages of activity: weight control, lower circulatory strain, diminished danger of diabetes, and expanded energy, just to give some examples. Yet, what might be said about the mental advantages of activity? From facilitating manifestations of wretchedness and uneasiness to keeping your memory sharp, there's no deficiency of mental advantages of activity. Regardless of whether you need the inspiration to get to the exercise center or to simply go for an energetic stroll, the five mental advantages of actual work beneath will make them tying up your shoe bands and taking off the entryway.

1. Help for discouragement and tension

Exercise is a logically demonstrated state of mind promoter, diminishing manifestations of both melancholy and tension. Active work kicks up endorphin levels, the body's wellknown "feel better" synthetically created by the mind and spinal string produces sensations of joy and rapture. Indeed, even moderate exercise over time can improve wretchedness and uneasiness, to such an extent that a few specialists suggest evaluating an activity routine for these conditions before going to drugs.

2. Diminished pressure

Another psychological advantage of activity is diminished feelings of anxiety, which can make us all more joyful. Expanding your pulse can really switch pressure prompted cerebrum harm by invigorating the creation of neurosurgeons like norepinephrine, which improve cognizance and mindset as well as improve suspecting obfuscated by unpleasant occasions. Exercise likewise powers the body's focal and thoughtful sensory systems to speak with each other, improving the body's general capacity to react to pressure.

3. Expanded confidence and self-assurance

From improving perseverance to getting more fit and expanding muscle tone, there's no deficiency of actual accomplishments that come to fruition from customary exercise. Every one of those accomplishments would all be able to amount to an astounding increase in confidence— and the certainty that accompanies it. You may not set out for better-fitting garments, slimmer physical make-up, and the capacity to climb a slope without getting short of breath. Customarily it occurs before you even acknowledge it. It's only one of the numerous advantages of actual work that support your body, psyche, and soul.

4. Better rest

If you experience difficulty getting a decent night's rest, exercise can assist with that, as well. Actual work builds internal heat levels, which can have quieting impacts on the psyche, prompting less sheep tallying and more shuteye. Exercise also directs your circadian mood, our bodies' underlying morning timer that controls when we feel tired and alert. (Albeit improved rest is a mental advantage of activity, rest specialists prescribe not practicing near sleep time.)

5. Cerebrum help

From building knowledge to reinforcing memory, the practice supports intellectual competence in various ways. Studies on mice and people show that cardiovascular exercise makes new synapses—an interaction called neurogenesis—and improves mind execution. It likewise forestalls intellectual decrease and cognitive decline by reinforcing the hippocampus, the piece of the cerebrum liable for memory and learning. Studies additionally demonstrate that actual work helps innovativeness and mental energy. So in case you're needing motivation, your large thought could be only a walk or run away.

PROVEN BENEFITS OF PHYSICAL ACTIVITY

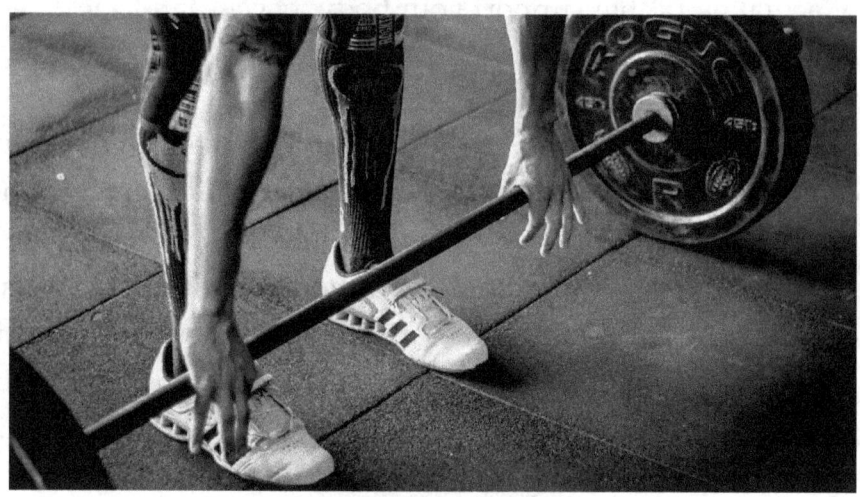

Physical activity refers to all the movement we carry out throughout the day, such as doing housework, bring in shopping, walking to work and doing exercise like playing a sport or going to the gym. Evidence continues to mount that being physically active can benefit both body and mind and reduce the risk of many diseases. Here are nine proven benefits of regular physical activity.

1. Keeps a sound body weight

2. Brings down pulse

3. Diminishes the danger of coronary illness

4. Brings down the danger of type 2 diabetes

5. Decreases the danger of specific malignancies

6. Expands muscle strength and capacity

7. Improves bone wellbeing and strength

8. Assists with advancing positive psychological wellness

9. Decreases the danger of dementia

1. Keeps a sound body weight

Low physical activity can increment somebody's danger of getting overweight or obese. 1 While practicing alone doesn't really prompt weight reduction; it can uphold effective weight decrease in blend with a balanced calorie-controlled eating regimen. Also, there is proof that actual daily work can help maintain solid body weight over time.

2. Brings down pulse

Hypertension (or hypertension) is a danger factor for some illnesses, particularly stroke and coronary illness. Standard active work can build your heart's solidarity, which lessens the exertion expected to siphon blood around the body. This declines the power on your conduits, diminishing circulatory strain. There is acceptable proof that normal actual work keeps up the sound circulatory strain.

3. Diminishes the danger of coronary illness

Normal exercise, especially aerobic workout, like lively strolling, running, and cycling, has diminished the danger of developing heart disease. This advantage is noticed for individuals of all body sizes. Individuals with overweight or obesity who are genuinely dynamic are undeniably less inclined to get coronary illness contrasted with the individuals who aren't.

4. Brings down the danger of type 2 diabetes

Exercise is known to help in the guideline of glucose levels and improves our body's affectability to insulin. Actual idleness, then again, has been reliably appeared to expand the danger of creating type 2 diabetes. Moreover, ordinary exercise is frequently prescribed to individuals with diabetes to help in their control of glucose levels.

5. Decreases the danger of specific malignancies

Cancer is a mysterious illness affected by numerous controllable (for example, smoking, unfortunate eating routine, high liquor utilization) and wild (for example, hereditary qualities, radiation, natural poisons) factors. Proof recommends that regular moderate to overwhelming activity can help diminish our danger of building up particular diseases, including colon, colorectal, lung and bosom malignant growths.

6. Expands muscle strength and capacity

Skeletal muscle serves numerous capacities, it looks after pose, controls development, and produces body heat. As we age, our bulk will diminish frequently because of a more stationary way of life. This deficiency of bulk can decrease our portability and increment our danger of falls and strong illnesses such as sarcopenia. 5 Regular workout, especially obstruction preparing (for example, lifting loads or bodyweight activities, squats and push-ups) can help improve muscle strength and versatility and diminish our danger of solid issues sarcopenia.

7. Improves bone wellbeing and strength

Weight-bearing exercise (e.g. running, dancing) and resistance training have been shown to improve bone density in adolescents and help maintain bone density in adulthood, reducing the risk of osteoporosis. This is particularly important for older adults and menopausal women as it can help to slow the natural loss of bone density that occurs with age.

8. Assists with advancing positive psychological wellness

Customary exercise has been appeared to positively affect our emotional wellness and mental well-being. 1 The precise system for which exercise benefits our psychological wellbeing isn't completely perceived. What is known is that ordinary exercise can advance the delivery of endorphins and help relieve stress and advance a sound rest design, which would all be able to cooperate to improve our state of mind. What's more, there is some proof to recommend that activity may even assistance in the treatment of gloom and other mental issues.

9. Decreases the danger of dementia

Regular exercise has been reliably appeared to secure against intellectual decline. 1 Although it is not completely seen how exercise diminishes psychological decay, ongoing proof recommends that the arrival of proteins known as neurotrophic factors probably play a significant role. These gainful variables help advance neuron development and fix, which help support ordinary intellectual functioning. 7 This may part of the way to clarify why more seasoned grownups who remain truly dynamic all through life have a much lower hazard of creating intellectual problems like dementia and Alzheimer's sickness.

How much physical activity should we do?

The World Health Organization recommends:

1. We do at least in any event 150 minutes of moderateintensity aerobic actual work consistently or, if nothing else, 75 minutes of vigorous-intensity aerobic active work consistently or a comparable mix of moderate and overwhelming force action.

2. Vigorous exercises ought to be acted in episodes of at any rate 10 minutes term.

3. For extra medical advantages, grown-ups should intend to expand their moderate-force high-impact active work to 300 minutes out of every week, or 150 minutes of incredible power high-impact active work each week, or a comparable mix of both moderate and positive power action.

4. Muscle-fortifying or anaerobic activities should be finished, including significant muscle gatherings (legs, hips, back, midsection, chest, shoulders, and arms) on at least 2 days every week.

It is prompted that individuals with earlier medical issues counsel well-being proficient before undertaking extra exercise.

Tips to expand your actual work

In the present occupied society, ordinary active work can be difficult to keep up and requires both time and exertion. Here are a few hints to help you increment your actual work levels:

- Set practical goals: committing to build your actual work is a significant initial step. Defining an objective (for example, get 10,000 stages each day) and arranging what you need to do to accomplish this objective (for example, plan to walk some portion of your drive) can help keep you engaged and submitted.

- Take the stairs: An simple approach to expand your dayby-day actual work is to use the stairwell rather than lifts or lifts at every possible opportunity.

- Get your companions involved: Exercise is better with companions, take a stab at joining a games group or going for a run or lively stroll with a companion.

- Walk a piece of your commute: Try getting off a stop early or stopping further away and strolling part of your drive.

- Take regular breaks from sitting: Many of us go through the more significant part of our days situated, be it busy working or home. Attempt to go for regular breaks to stroll around, stretch your legs, and try not to sit for significant stretches.

- Make it fun: Exercise shouldn't be an errand, similar to eating a solid adjusted eating regimen. In the event that we detest it, we will not have the option to keep it up for long. Attempt to discover a movement that you appreciate and can adhere to the long haul.

The Body, Mind and Spirit: The benefits of Exercises
Even though it might assist you with getting thinner and forestall persistent illnesses like diabetes, hypertension and cardiovascular infection, practice likewise benefits the brain and soul. Did you realize that normal exercise can lift your mood, fight depression, lessen anxiety and slow the psychological decline that accompanies age? The advantages of customary exercise appear to be unending, and we can assist you with appreciating these advantages.

On the off chance that you are feeling down, practice is most likely the exact opposite thing you need to do. However, a few examinations have affirmed that active work can:

- discharge endorphins and other "feel better" mind synthetics that can ease melancholy

- occupy you in a positive path from a pattern of negative musings and feelings that add to the tension

- increase positive social association

- boost confidence levels

Studies have discovered that activity is more than a momentary mindset lifter. Information proposes that dynamic individuals are less discouraged than idle individuals and that regular exercise can be a powerful intervention for those experiencing gloom.

On the off chance that that is an insufficient inspiration to be all the more truly dynamic, examines have also tracked down those stationary individuals who take up another activity routine to curb the pace of mental decline that accompanies age. Genuinely dynamic, more established grown-ups have stronger recall and thinking abilities.

Top Benefits of Strength Training

While all types of exercise can improve your well-being, strength training is unquestionably the most beneficial.

Power training (like lunges, squats, push-ups, and arm curls) will help you look and feel your best, from increased strength and endurance to better bone health and regulated body fat.

"My personal favorite strength exercises are deadlifts or something explosive like power cleans," says Amanda Vargas, a Beachbody fitness expert. "I really enjoy incorporating something that challenges balance, whether it's using unstable equipment like a stability ball or doing some exercises single-legged or single-armed," she continues.

1. Better Sleep Quality

Muscle building and strength training, according to the Sleep Foundation, will "improve the quality of sleep, as well as help you fall asleep quicker and wake up less often during the night."

"Better sleep quality has a lot of benefits in terms of a person's overall wellness," Vargas says. These advantages include, among other things, a lower risk of illness, an improved mood, and weight control.

2. Decrease Stress

All of us are experiencing increased tension and anxiety these days. Power training workouts are an excellent way to combat tension.

Vargas claims that "exercise endorphins contribute to relaxation." It may also aid in the reduction of depressive symptoms and the stabilization of your overall mood. A winwin situation!

3. Does Meathead Construct Your Brain?

It's almost of a brainiac. "Lifting weights promotes more than just muscle development. "Studies show that it can potentially activate brain connections and improve cognitive function," says famous Trainer Joey Wilkins.

4. May Reduce the Risk of Dementia

"Resistance training tends to help thicken the gray matter in a region of the brain that is often affected in early Alzheimer's disease, and it also appears to help develop brain cells," Wilkins says.

If you have a family history of dementia or Alzheimer's, strength training might be particularly beneficial to you.

5. Increases Endurance

While you might not think cardio and strength training go hand in hand, Wilkins explains that building stronger muscles "will actually help your cardio sessions be more effective by way of more force development and work economy."

Runners, don't skimp on the bicep twists, squats, and deadlifts.

6. Improved Posture and Injury Prevention

According to Vargas, the advantages of strength training include improved posture and also injury prevention because it improves the strength of the body's tendons and ligaments (aka connective tissues). This could be particularly helpful if you sit hunched over at a desk all day!

7. Lowers the risk of osteoporosis

Though strength training has advantages for both men and women. Strength training over a man's life will increase bone density and keep her bones strong," Vargas says.

THE BEACH BODY WORKOUT

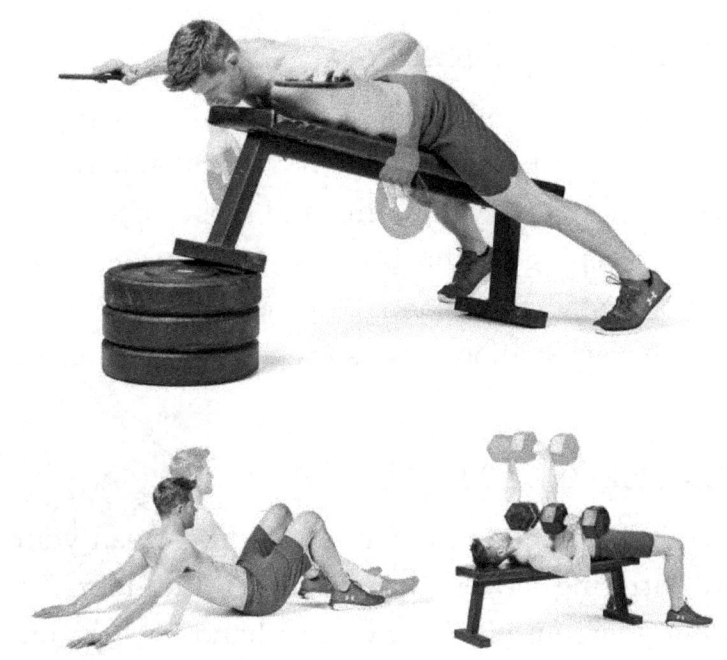

The Warm-up

Utilize these drills to prime your body for every exercise meeting.

1. Descending Dog to Spider Lunge

Start in pushup position, feet shoulder-width separated. Keeping your legs straight, raise your butt; attempt to remain adjusted from middle to arms. Hold. Get back to the pushup position. Without moving your left leg, bring your correct foot outside your correct hand. Get back to the beginning; rehash the grouping on the opposite side. That is 1 rep; complete 2 arrangements of 10.

2. Superman to Floor Angel

Falsehood facedown on the floor with your arms expanded. All the while, fix your glutes, raise your legs, and fix your back muscles as you raise your arms and upper chest. This is the beginning. Keeping up this position, fan your arms in reverse. Attempt to contact your hands together on your back. Get back to the beginning position. That is 1 rep; complete 2 arrangements of 10.

3. Youngster's Pose to Reach and Rotate

Stoop with your enormous toes contacting. Lean your middle forward, arriving at your hands out on the floor. This is the beginning position. Lift your correct hand. String your correct arm under your left armpit. Get back to the beginning. That is 1 rep; complete 2 arrangements of 10 for every side.

4. Speed Jacks

Remain with your arms at your sides, feet together. Begin doing bouncing jacks, however, as opposed to keeping a casual speed, move your arms and feet as quickly as possible. Keep at it for 30 seconds; at that point, rest for 30 seconds. Work through 2 rounds.

The Schedule

DAY 1 PAIRED SETS

1 DB snatch + 3 Pushup, 2 DB front squat + 4 Inverted Row, 5 Burpee

Do alternating 30-second intervals of moves 1 and 3 for the time listed below. Rest 3 minutes. Do 2 and 4 the same way. Finish up with a 4-minute Tabata (work for 20 seconds, rest 10) of move 5.

DAY 2 PAIRED SETS

6 Chinup + 7 Broad jumps, 8 Push press + 9 Jump lunge, 10 Lateral shuffle

Do alternating 30-second intervals of moves 6 and 7 for the time listed below. Rest 3 minutes. Do 8 and 9 the same way. Finish up with a 4-minute Tabata (work for 20 seconds, rest 10) of move 10.

PAIRED SET WORKOUTS

- Week 1: 12 minutes
- Week 2: 14 minutes
- Week 3: 16 minutes
- Week 4: 18 minutes

DAY 3 REST/CARDIO

DAY 4 INTERVALS

1 DB snatch + 3 Pushup + 2 DB front squat + 4

Inverted Row, 5 Burpee

Do moves 1, 3, 2, and 4 in that order. Spend 6 straight minutes on each, following the rest/reps guide below. Rest 2 minutes between moves. Finish up with a 4-minute Tabata of move 5.

DAY 5 INTERVALS

6 Chinup + 7 Broad jump + 8 Push press + 9 Jump lunge, 10 Lateral shuffle

Do moves 6, 7, 8, and 9 in order. Spend 6 straight minutes on each, following the rest/reps guide below. Rest 2 minutes between moves. Finish up with a 4-minute Tabata of move 10.

INTERVAL WORKOUTS

- Week 1: 30 seconds on, 30 off
- Week 2: 40 seconds on, 20 off
- Week 3: 45 seconds on, 15 off
- Week 4: 50 seconds on, 10 off

DAY 6 REST/CARDIO

DAY 7 REST/CARDIO

The Moves

1. Hand weight Snatch

Hold a free weight in your correct hand at mid-shin level with your knees twisted and a slight pivot in your hips. Pull the load up as you violently fix your knees and hips. (In the event that you remain on your pussyfoots, that is OK.) As the weight arrives at shoulder tallness, expand your correct arm straight up. That is 1 rep. Start with your correct arm on the initially set; switch back and forth between arms each set after that.

2. Hand weight Front Squat

Remain with hand weights against the meatiest pieces of your shoulders. Curve at your knees, bringing down your middle until your thighs are corresponding to the floor. Get back to standing. That is 1 rep.

3. Pushup

Expect a pushup position, your hands marginally past shoulder width, feet together, and center tight. Twist at your elbows to bring down your middle an inch from the floor; at that point, push back up. Consistently, keep your lower arms opposite to the floor and your center as close as could be expected. That is 1 rep.

4. Transformed line

Hang a suspension mentor from a pullup bar, so its handles are about abdomen high. Lie under it, your chest lined up with the handles and legs straight. Get the handles utilizing an impartial grasp, and pull your middle to the handles. Lower your middle. That is 1 rep. (Excessively hard? Set the handles somewhat higher and accept a place that is nearer to standing.)

5. Burpee

Start in a standing position. Pivot at your hips, set your hands on the floor, kick your feet back in a wide position, and lower your chest to the floor. Get up as fast as you can by kicking your feet forward and standing. Wrap up by bouncing straight up. That is 1 rep.

6. Chinup

Swing from a bar utilizing an underhand, shoulder-width hold. Crush your shoulder bones, fix your center, and pull your chest to the bar (or as near it as you can get). Gradually lower yourself back to hanging, keeping up slight strain in your center back. That is 1 rep.

7. Wide Jump

Remain with your feet about shoulder-width separated and knees somewhat bowed. Pivot at your hips, twist all the more profoundly with your knees and toss your arms in reverse. Presently toss your arms forward and take a major jump. Land with your feet still separated. Your knees ought to be marginally twisted to pad your arrival. At that point, retreat to the beginning line. That is 1 rep.

8. Push Press

Stand holding hand weights at your shoulders, your feet about shoulder-width separated. Your elbows ought to be twisted, and palms are confronting one another. Keeping your center tight, twist your knees marginally; at that point, dangerously fix them. Utilize the energy to press the free weights over your shoulders until your arms are straight. Try not to curve your back as you do this. Lower the loads back to your shoulders. That is 1 rep.

9. Bounce Lunge

Expect a stunning position, your left foot forward. Curve the two knees and lower your middle until your left thigh is corresponding to the floor and your correct shin is near the floor. Violently remain back up. As you do this, bounce and shift your feet so your correct foot arrives before your left. That is 1 rep. At the point when you land, you should as of now be in a situation for the following rep.

10. Parallel Shuffle

Remain with your feet about shoulder-width separated, knees twisted. Rapidly mix 10 stages to one side and afterward 10 stages to one side. Attempt to keep your chest up, and don't allow your feet to cross before one another as you do this. Consider remaining low to the ground. (Short on space? Make fewer moves to each side; simply ensure you're rearranging the whole time).

Summer is practically here. So on the off chance that you need an exceptionally viable preparing plan to barrage yourself into fit physique shape, you're in the perfect spot.

This four-week plan has been intended to convey the greatest bang for your back. To this end, it's part into two fortnight-long "blocks": the principal square will establish the frameworks of greater, more grounded muscles and start the way toward stripping away fat, while the second is a fullscale attack on the iron to constrain your body to add slender, hard bulk while consuming

the rest of your muscle to fat ratio stores for fuel. So, it will significantly change what you look like – and feel – without your shirt on.

Just read the directions beneath, at that point, begin on the arrangement. It's not difficult to follow, however it will require devotion and center from you to get the ideal outcomes. Give it all that you have and perceive how you can improve your body in only one month.

The Training Plan Explained

The hypothesis

The arrangement contains two squares. The first has four meetings per week: chest and arms; legs and delts; back and arms; and chest and delts. It implies you're preparing your significant chest area muscles double seven days, a highrecurrence approach that will change your body quickly.

Super beginning

The exercises for the primary fortnight of the arrangement start underneath. In this initial fourteen-day block, every exercise has six moves: the initial two are proceeded as straight sets, at that point the third and fourth move are done as a superset, just like the fifth and 6th moves. Follow the request precisely.

Gain train
==========

This extreme focus approach implies you'll assemble muscle and consume fat. Do the activities all together, adhering to the sets, reps, beat and rest periods itemized.

The beat code alludes to the number of seconds taken to finish each piece of the activity. Taking the seat press for instance, the main digit alludes to how you require to bring down the weight, the subsequent digit how long to stop at the lower part of the lift, the third how since a long time ago taken to lift the weight, lastly the fourth digit alludes to how long you stop at the highest point of the development.

In week two the exercises are something similar, then again, actually some key factors have been changed to keep your body comp acquires coming. Jump to week two of square one.

Huge changes
============

In the last fortnight of the arrangement, the meetings have been changed to stun your body into developing. However much bulk as could be expected while stripping away the greatest measure of fat. There are four meetings: chest and rear arm muscles, legs and abs; back and biceps, and chest and delts. Jump to impede two, week one.

Solid completion
================

In this second square, every one of the moves is made as straight sets so you can zero in on lifting as hefty as possible while keeping up the great structure and hitting the objective rep tally.

For the last week, the key factors have changed, so you finish as large and lean as possible. Jump to impede two, week two.

Way of life Tips

Help your body add most extreme muscle while burning however much paunch fat as could reasonably be expected by receiving these four better-body propensities.

Drink more

Water, that is. Remaining hydrated has more than once been appeared to improve physical and mental prosperity and execution. Exploration has discovered that individuals who drank more water felt less exhausted, wise to center, and experienced improved mindset – all factors that advance a feeling of prosperity. Focus on at any rate two liters per day, and convey a water bottle around with you so it's not difficult to continue to drink the entire day.

Be careful

Zeroing in on what's going on at the time can bring down your feelings of anxiety and improve inspiration. In case you're new to care, start with being more careful at eating times. This implies is having suppers from the TV, your telephone and different interruptions, so you center around the demonstration of eating and how it affects you. It will make you more cognizant about the thing you're placing in your body and forestall over-eating.

Eat your greens

Eating more veg is the absolute most significant propensity to embrace for more noteworthy wellbeing. Veg is loaded with nutrients, minerals, fiber and different mixtures, for example, phytochemicals that have various wellbeing boosting characteristics. Eat around two clench hand estimated bit of veggies with each dinner, close by a palmsized bit of great protein, and you'll change your body quicker than you expected.

Rest further

Great quality rest is crucial for building muscle and getting fit, so put your telephone and PC to bed at any rate 45 minutes before you need to head to sleep to improve your odds of nodding off and staying unconscious. These screens radiate blue light, which is a similar frequency as day break light, as is deciphered by your cerebrum as a sign that it's an ideal opportunity to awaken and get dynamic. Turn every one of your screens off, at that point turn in.

Block 1 - Week 1

Monday Workout: Chest And Arms

1. Bench press

Falsehood level on a seat, holding a bar with a shoulderwidth grasp. Plant your feet on the floor and tense your muscles. Lower the bar until it contacts your chest, at that point, press it back up effectively.

2. Cable get over

Stand tall in a link machine, holding a D-handle in each hand connected to the high pulley. Keeping your chest up and center propped, bring your hands down in a smooth curve to meet before your body. Hold briefly, at that point get back to the beginning.

3. Incline dumbbell shoulder press

Falsehood level on a grade seat, holding a free weight in each hand at chest tallness. Plant your feet on the floor and get your body tight. Press the loads straight up, so your arms are straight; at that point, lower them leveled out.

4. Incline biceps twist

Sit on a grade seat, holding a free weight in each hand with your palms confronting advances and your elbows tight to your sides. Keeping your elbows there, twist the loads up to bear stature. Press your biceps at the top, at that point bring down the loads.

5. Cable biceps twist

Stand tall before a link machine, holding a bar handle connected to the lower pulley with palms looking up. Keeping your chest up and elbows tight to your sides, twist your hands up to bear tallness. Crush your biceps at the top, at that point lower.

6. Cable rear arm muscles push down

Stand tall before a link machine, holding a bar handle appended to the high pulley with palms looking down. Keeping your chest up and elbows tight to your sides, press your hands down to fix your arms, at that point gradually get back to the beginning.

Wednesday Workout: Legs And Delts

1. Back squat

Stand tall, holding a hand weight across the rear of your shoulders. Keeping your chest up and your entire body tense, twist your knees to crouch as low as possible yet don't allow your knees to roll inwards. Push through your heels to remain back up.

2. Overhead press

Stand tall, holding a hand weight across the front of your chest with an overhand grasp. Keeping your chest up and center drew in, press the bar straightforwardly overhead so your arms are straight. Lower it leveled out to get back to the beginning.

3. Leg augmentation

Position yourself accurately on the machine with the cushioned bar against the lower part of your shins. Keeping your chest area tense, raise your feet to fix your legs. Respite at the top with your quads drew in, at that point lower back to the beginning.

4. Hamstring twist

Position yourself effectively on the machine with the cushioned bar against the rear of your lower legs. Keeping your chest area tense, push your feet down to twist your legs.

Interruption at the top with your hamstrings drew in, at that point lower back to the beginning.

5. Seated dumbbell overhead press

Sit on an upstanding seat, holding a free weight in each hand at shoulder tallness. Keeping your chest up and center supported, press the loads straightforwardly overhead so your arms are straight. Gradually lower back to the beginning.

6. Seated dumbbell lateral raise

Sit on an upstanding seat, holding a light free weight in each hand by your sides with a slight twist in your elbows. Keeping your chest up and center propped, raise the loads out to bear stature, driving with your elbows. Return gradually to the beginning.

Friday Workout: Back And Arms

1. Bent-over column

Hold a hand weight with a shoulder-width grasp, bowing your knees marginally. Curve at the hips until you're at generally 45° to the floor. Pull the bar up to contact your sternum, at that point lower leveled out. In case you're moving your chest area to move the bar, the weight's excessively hefty.

2. Lat drawdown

Position yourself at the machine with a shoulder-width overhand hold on the bar. Keeping your chest up and abs supported, pull the bar down, driving with your elbows. Stand firm on the base foothold briefly, at that point get back to the beginning.

3. Seated link line

Sit on the machine, holding a twofold grasp link connection in two hands. Keeping your chest up, line your hands in towards your body, driving with your elbows. Delay at the top position, at that point get back to the beginning.

4. Underhand lat pull-down

Position yourself at the machine with a restricted underhand grasp on the bar. Keeping your chest up and abs propped, pull the bar down, driving with your elbows. Stand firm on the base footing briefly, at that point get back to the beginning.

5. Cable straight-arm pull-down

Stand tall, confronting the link machine and holding a straight bar handle with two hands. Keeping your arms straight, pull the bar down towards your thighs in a smooth curve. Interruption at the base, at that point, turns around the development back to the beginning.

6. Cable rear arm muscles push down

Stand tall, confronting the link machine and holding a straight bar handle with palms looking down. Keeping your chest up and elbows tight to your sides, press your hands down to fix your arms; at that point, gradually get back to the beginning.

Saturday Workout: Chest And Delts

1. Incline seat press

Untruth level on a grade seat, holding a hand weight with a shoulder-width grasp. Plant your feet on the floor and tense your muscles. Lower the bar until it contacts your chest, at that point press it back up effectively.

2. Incline dumbbell flye

Lie on a slope seat, holding two free weights straight over your chest with straight arms. Curve your elbows marginally, at that point bring down your hands out to the sides until you feel a stretch across your chest. Press your pecs to get back to the beginning.

3. EZ-Bar upright line

Stand tall, holding an EZ-bar with a shoulder-width overhand grasp. Keeping your chest up and center supported, column the bar up to jawline tallness, driving with your elbows. Interruption at the top, at that point, bring down the bar back to the beginning leveled out.

4. Dumbbell lateral raise

Stand tall, holding a light free weight in each hand by your sides with a slight curve in your elbows. Keeping your chest up and center supported, raise the loads out to bear stature, driving with your elbows, at that point return gradually to the beginning.

5. Dumbbell draw over

Untruth level on a seat, holding a free weight with two hands over your chest with straight arms. Lower the load behind your head leveled out, keeping your arms straight, at that point raise it back to the beginning position.

6. Press-up

Get down on the ground with your legs and arms straight, your hands under your shoulders, and your body in an orderly fashion from head to heels. Draw in your abs and twist your elbows to bring down your chest towards the floor, at that point press back up intensely.

Square 1 - Week 2

With week 1 clinched, you ought to feel and looking great. You'll have effectively seen your T-shirt sleeves feeling somewhat tighter and perhaps climbed an indent on your belt. Yet, presently's not an opportunity to kick back and celebrate – it's an ideal opportunity to push on harder to speed up your outcomes.

In this second seven-day stretch of the arrangement, you'll do similar exercises in a similar request as in the principal week. Every one of the moves of every exercise is the equivalent as well. This isn't us being languid: because you are presently acquainted with this daily schedule, you can assault every meeting harder to make the correct improvement for your body to expand the measure of muscle it can construct and fat it can consume.

Also, there's one major distinction in this week to make the exercises harder (and subsequently more powerful). There's an extra set for the initial four moves of every meeting – so you'll complete four arrangements of moves 1, 2, 3A, and 3B. Remain on track and keep the confidence – this is a major week and you need to get after it from the primary rep of each set.

Monday Workout: Chest And Arms

Exercise	Sets	Reps	Tempo	Rest
1 Bench press	4	12	2010	60sec
2 Cable cross-over	4	12	2011	60sec
3 Incline dumbbell press	4	12	2010	30sec
4 Incline biceps curl	4	12	2011	60sec
5 Cable biceps curl	3	15	2011	30sec
6 Cable triceps press	3	15	2010	60sec

Wednesday Workout: Legs And Delts

Exercise	Sets	Reps	Tempo	Rest
1 Squat	4	12	2010	60sec
2 Overhead press	4	12	2010	60sec
3 Leg extension	4	12	2011	30sec
4 Hamstring curl	4	12	2011	60sec
5 Seated overhead press	3	15	2010	30sec

6 Seated lateral raise	3	15	2010	60sec

Friday Workout: Back And Arms

Exercise	Sets	Reps	Tempo	Rest
1 Bent-over row	4	12	2011	60sec
2 Lat pull-down	4	12	2011	60sec
3A Seated row	4	12	2011	30sec
3 Underhand lat pull-down	4	12	2011	60sec
4 Straight-arm pull-down	3	15	2011	30sec
5 Cable triceps press	3	15	2011	60sec

Saturday Workout: Chest And Delts

Exercise	Sets	Reps	Tempo	Rest
1 Incline bench press	4	12	2010	60sec
2 Incline dumbbell flye	4	12	2011	60sec
3 EZ-bar upright row	4	12	2011	30sec
4 Dumbbell lateral raise	4	12	2011	60sec
5 Dumbbell pull-over	3	15	2010	30sec

6 Press-up   3   15   2010   60sec

Square 2: Week 1

Monday Workout: Chest And Triceps

1. Incline seat press

Falsehood level on a grade seat, holding a bar with a shoulder-width grasp. Plant your feet on the floor and tense your muscles. Lower the bar until it contacts your chest, at that point press it back up intensely.

2. Triceps plunge

Grasp equal bars with straight arms and your legs crossed behind you. Keeping your chest up and center supported, bring down your body by bowing your elbows until they're at 90°. Press back dependent upon getting back to the beginning.

3. Dumbbell seat press

Falsehood level on a level seat, holding a free weight in each hand at chest stature. Plant your feet on the floor and tense your muscles. Press the loads straight up so your arms are straight, at that point lower they leveled out.

4. Cable get over

Stand tall in a link machine, holding a D-handle in each hand appended to the high pulley. Keeping your chest up and center propped, bring your hands down in a smooth curve to meet before your body. Hold briefly, at that point get back to the beginning.

    5. One-arm link press

Stand tall with your back to a link machine, holding a Dhandle in one hand. Keeping your chest up and center supported, press your hand advances until your arm is straight. Turn around the transition to the beginning and rehash for every one of the reps to switch arms.

    6. Cable rear arm muscles push down

Stand tall, confronting the link machine and holding a straight bar handle with palms looking down. Keeping your chest up and elbows tight to your sides, press your hands down to fix your arms, at that point gradually get back to the beginning.

Wednesday Workout: Legs And Abs

    1. Back squat

Stand tall, holding a hand weight across the rear of your shoulders. Keeping your chest up and your entire body tense, twist your knees to crouch as low as possible yet don't allow your knees to roll inwards. Push through your heels to remain back up.

    2. Romanian deadlift

Stand tall with your feet shoulder-width separated, holding a free weight with an overhand grasp. With a slight curve in your knees, pivot advances from the hips and lower the bar until you feel a stretch in your hamstrings. Switch the transition to the beginning.

3. Leg expansion

Position yourself accurately on the machine with the cushioned bar against the lower part of your shins. Keeping your chest area tense, raise your feet to fix your legs. Interruption at the top with your quads drew in, at that point lower back to the beginning.

4. Hamstring twist

Position yourself effectively on the machine with the cushioned bar against the rear of your lower legs. Keeping your chest area tense, push your feet down to twist your legs. Delay at the top with your hamstrings drew in, at that point lower back to the beginning.

5. Hanging knee raise

Dangle from a bar with your legs straight and abs supported. Utilize your lower abs to draw your knees up towards your middle, at that point bring down your feet until your legs are straight. Keep strain on your center all through.

6. Crunch

Falsehood level on your back with your knees bowed and feet level on the floor, and fold your arms over your chest (or contact your fingers to your sanctuaries). Draw in your abs, at that point raise your middle off the floor without straining your neck. Lower back to the beginning.

Friday Workout: Back And Biceps

1. Hammer-grip chin-up

Grasp the handles with palms confronting and hang with your body straight. Support your abs and glutes and connect with your lats, at that point pull up until your jawline is over your hands. Interruption at the top, at that point lower yourself back to the beginning, leveled out.

2. Wide-hold lat pull-down

Position yourself at the machine, holding the bar with hands as widely separated as could really be expected. Keeping your chest up and abs propped, pull the bar down, driving with your elbows. Stand firm on the base footing briefly, at that point get back to the beginning.

3. Prone free weight column

Untruth chest down on a grade seat, holding a free weight in each hand. Keeping your chest against the seat, column the loads up, driving with your elbows. Stand firm on the top footing briefly, at that point bring down the loads back to the beginning.

4. Prone hand weight flye

Falsehood chest down on a slope seat holding a light free weight in each hand. Keeping your chest against the seat, raise the loads out to the sides, driving with your elbows. Stand firm on the top foothold briefly, at that point bring down the loads back to the beginning.

5. Seated link column

Sit on the machine, holding a twofold grasp link connection in two hands. Keeping your chest up, column your hands in towards your body, driving with your elbows. Interruption at the top position, at that point, get back to the beginning.

6. Incline biceps twist

Sit on a slope seat, holding a free weight in each hand with your palms confronting advances and your elbows tight to your sides. Keeping your elbows there, twist the loads up to bear stature. Crush your biceps at the top, at that point bring down the loads.

Saturday Workout: Delts And Abs

1. Seated dumbbell overhead press

Sit on an upstanding seat, holding a free weight in each hand at shoulder tallness. Keeping your chest up and center supported, press the loads straightforwardly overhead so your arms are straight. Gradually lower back to the beginning.

2. Seated dumbbell lateral raise

Sit on an upstanding seat, holding a light free weight in each hand by your sides with a slight curve in your elbows. Keeping your chest up and center supported, raise the loads out to bear tallness, driving with your elbows. Return gradually to the beginning.

3. EZ-bar upright line

Stand tall, holding an EZ-bar with a shoulder-width overhand grasp. Keeping your chest up and center supported, column the bar up to jawline tallness, driving with your elbows. Interruption at the top, at that point, bring down the bar back to the beginning leveled out.

4. Weighted seat crunch

Untruth level on a seat with your knees twisted and feet level on the floor, holding a free weight in two hands over your chest. Draw in your abs, at that point raise your middle of the seat without straining your neck. Lower back to the beginning.

5. Hanging knee raise

Swing from a bar with your legs straight and abs supported. Utilize your lower abs to draw your knees up towards your middle, at that point bring down your feet until your legs are straight. Keep strain on your center all through.

6. Plank

Get into position, supporting yourself on your lower arms with your elbows under your shoulders. Draw in your abs, at that point raise your hips so your body frames a straight line from head to heels. Stand firm on the present situation and don't allow your hips to hang.

Square 2 - Week 2

As we clarified toward the beginning of this exercise plan, everything changed after the main fortnight – the subsequent square contains meetings that hit distinctive body bunches in an alternate request utilizing various moves. That is because you need to shake things up routinely to hold your body back from sinking into its usual range of familiarity so you can add huge measures of fit bulk and make the correct conditions for consuming stomach fat so those abs are uncovered.

What's more, similarly as with the second seven-day stretch of square 1, there are some critical changes in the second seven-day stretch of square 2 as well: in particular that you'll do additional reps for each set of each move. In certain examples, you will actually want to lift a similar load as in the primary week and work your muscles significantly harder, however for certain moves, you may have to decrease the load to hit the objective rep check. Focus on hitting the reps and rhythm focus over lifting as substantial as conceivable because that is the thing that gets the best outcomes.

Monday Workout: Chest And Triceps

Exercise	Sets	Reps	Tempo	Rest
1 Incline bench press	4	10	3010	60sec
2 Triceps dip	4	10	3010	60sec
3 Dumbbell bench press	4	12	3010	60sec
4 Cable cross-over	4	12	3011	60sec

5 One-arm cable press	4	15	3011	60sec
6 Cable triceps press	4	15	3011	60sec

Wednesday Workout: Legs And Abs

Exercise	Sets	Reps	Tempo	Rest
1 Squat	4	10	3010	60sec
2 Romanian deadlift	4	10	3010	60sec
3 Leg extension	4	12	3011	60sec
4 Hamstring curl	4	12	3011	60sec
5 Hanging knee raise	4	15	3011	60sec
6 Crunch	4	15	3011	60sec

Friday Workout: Back And Biceps

Exercise	Sets	Reps	Tempo	Rest
1 Hammer-grip chin-up	4	10	3011	60sec
2 Wide-grip lat pull-down	4	10	3011	60sec
3 Prone dumbbell row	4	12	3011	60sec
4 Prone dumbbell flye	4	12	3011	60sec

5 Seated row	4	15	3011	60sec
6 Incline dumbbell curl	4	15	3011	60sec

Saturday Workout: Delts And Abs

Exercise	Sets	Reps	Tempo	Rest
1 Seated overhead press	4	10	3010	60sec
2 Seated lateral raise	4	10	3011	60sec
3 EZ-bar upright row	4	12	3011	60sec
4 Weighted bench crunch	4	12	3011	60sec
5 Hanging knee raise	4	15	3011	60sec
6 Plank	4	60sec	N/A	60sec

When a warm climate strikes, will your body be seashore prepared? On the off chance that you will likely get an ideal body, you've gone to the correct spot. This rundown of seven eating routines and wellness tips will assist you with getting a body you'll be glad for flaunting when shirts fall off. We should not burn through any additional time: Here's how you need to help a lean body.

1.   Everything begins with your eating routine. Diet – not wellness – has the greatest impact on whether you'll shed the

important fat to get the ideal fit physique. You can work out 20 times each day, however, it won't help you very much if your eating regimen isn't satisfactory. Other than many products of the soil, a solid eating routine should comprise entire grains and lean protein. Most food varieties that are high in these supplements are low in calories and fat. Likewise, you ought to be taking a men's multivitamin to fill any wholesome holes in your eating plan. At last, you need to make a calorie shortfall to consume fat, so slice calories every week to invigorate weight reduction.

2. Drink enough water. Experts currently propose you drink in any event 10 glasses of water to remain adequately hydrated for the duration of the day – and surprisingly more, in case you're genuinely dynamic. You don't really need to drink that much water – you can likewise get water from products of the soil sources like a men's post-exercise shake. Deficient water admission can prompt drying out, which can bring about muscle cramps and different issues.

3. Have 5-6 dinners a day. Eating more modest suppers for the duration of the day rather than three major suppers can help you control hunger better, which thus may prompt more proficient weight reduction. You shouldn't make every one of these dinners a 5-course issue; a men's whey protein shake or a little pack of trail blend tallies toward this aggregate. On the off chance that you eat huge segments at each feast, you will accomplish more damage than anything else.

4.   Perform cardiovascular exercise, in any event, multiple times a week. Aerobic movement, for example, running or swimming, assists individuals with getting thinner and get a fit figure. Discover what activities and settings turn out best for you. Perhaps you're the kind of individual who leans towards the treadmill at the rec center as opposed to a plunge in an outside pool. Notwithstanding what you pick, make sure to take a men's pre-exercise supplement to help exercise execution for quicker, apparent outcomes.

5.   Perform strength preparing in any event double a week. This is pivotal for individuals who need a conditioned body. If everything you do is cardio, you will wind up with free skin and basically no muscle tone. Try to work the entirety of your significant muscle gatherings – don't simply zero in on alluring muscles like your arms. You ought to likewise focus on your legs and back, which are frequently disregarded. Consider a men's creatine supplement for more muscle strength and force; creatine gives your muscles additional energy for anaerobic exercise like weight preparation.

6.   Get a lot of sleep. Although a few groups can run on just five hours of rest, focus on 7-9 hours. A few examinations recommend that an absence of rest may add to weight acquire – also an arrangement of other medical issues. In case you're experiencing difficulty dozing, begin tallying some sheep or do some essential breathing activities to take your psyche off things. Some of the time, a snarling stomach can hold us back from nodding off. In the event that evening hunger is

influencing your sleep, blend a whey protein shake to top you off without rounding you out.

THE BEST BEACH BODY DIET

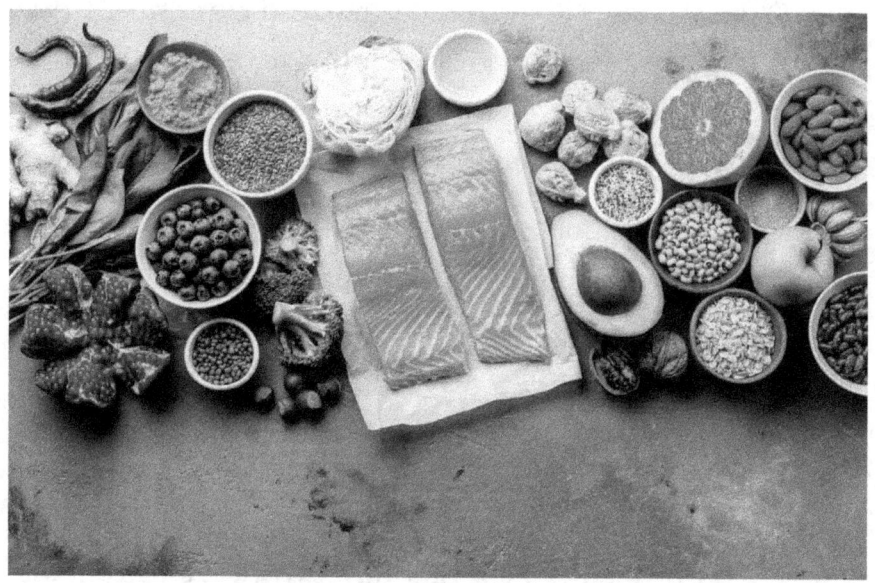

The best way to lose weight and see your abs is to eat fewer calories than you are now. Nothing else, not weight lifting, cardio, or vitamins, will compensate for failing to follow this basic law. That is everything there is to it. But, if you can postpone your pizza and beer day for the next six weeks, keep reading because we'll show you how to get a six-pack before summer ends.

It all comes down to calories.

To lose weight, you must eat more calories than you consume — but this does not imply that you can do so by exercise. "Exercise by itself is pretty useless for weight loss," Eric Ravussin, Ph.D., a weight-loss specialist and professor at the Pennington

Biomedical Research Center in Baton Rouge, LA, famously told The New York Times. He eventually made the argument that people not only eat more calories than they can burn, but that the additional strain of exercise increases appetite, making it much easier to absorb the calories they've worked off.

According to Mayo Clinic research, a 160-pound person doing high-impact aerobic exercise will only burn 533 calories in an hour. (It's worth noting that most people aren't capable of maintaining an extreme pace for that long.) Consider that a balanced dinner consisting of four ounces of skinless chicken breast and one cup of rice has 385 calories. That's right: If you eat one light meal, you'll be a stone's throw away from recouping the calories you burned during that day's workout—assuming the workout was long and incredibly vigorous in the first place.

So, if you can't build a caloric deficit through exercise (at least not without a lot of it, marathon runners excluded), you must do it through diet. To begin, multiply your current body weight by 12 to determine how many calories you should eat per day. If you're incredibly overweight, base your diet on the bodyweight you want to achieve. So, if you're 220 pounds but recall feeling and looking your best when you were 190, start eating 2,300 calories a day (190 x 12, rounded up for simplicity).

Take note of the macros.

Working out does not burn enough calories to affect fat loss on its own, but it does help muscle mass, allowing for a healthier, more attractive, leaner body. To get the most out of your weight training, you must eat the right mix of macronutrients. Protein is the most important component of muscle tissue, so consume enough of it—aim for one gram per pound of bodyweight (or target weight, as explained above).

Fat, while being calorically dense, plays an important role in developing hormones such as testosterone, so while it must be held relatively low to help generate the caloric deficit we're looking for, it can't be eliminated entirely. Eat 0.4 grams of fat per pound of body weight—a 200-pound man will consume 80 grams a day. The majority of your fat intake should be a byproduct of the protein-rich foods you consume.

Now we're down to carbs, and while there's been a lot of debate about their position in a fat-loss diet in recent years, there shouldn't be. "You need a moderate amount of carbs to help the fueling and recovery demands of high-intensity, anaerobic-based training," says Nate Miyaki, C.S.S.N., a San Francisco-based amateur bodybuilder diet coach, and author. Extreme low-carb diets, especially those that substitute bacon, cheese, and other fatty foods for carbs, do not function in the long run and (surprise!) do not promote optimal health. "Training fails when you're on low carbs," says Bryan Krahn, C.S.C.S., a personal trainer in New York City. "If your carbohydrate intake is extremely low, you will experience a decrease in metabolic rate. It's a sledgehammer approach to weight loss that's unnecessary; simply reduce your caloric intake."

As with protein, strive for one gram of carbs per pound of body weight. Please keep in mind that these figures are just a starting point. They should encourage you to lose one or two pounds a week at first (more if you're heavier), but if your weight loss stalls for more than a week, reduce your calories and recalculate your numbers. Reduce to 11 calories per pound at first, then to 10 later. It is important to note that losing more than two pounds per week does not result in greater fat loss. Extreme weight loss is more likely to be from water or, worse, muscle fat, so a steady yet gradual diet is best. Reports of people who have lost weight more quickly cannot be believed.

Consume just healthy foods.

Animal foods are the best sources of protein because they contain all of the amino acids needed by the body to perform all of its functions, including muscle building. Chicken, fish, eggs, lean beef, and turkey should be part of your daily diet. Protein powder supplements are another choice. A three-tofour-ounce portion of lean meat is around the size and thickness of your palm and contains 20–25 grams of protein and five grams of fat or less (if you're not sure, look up the nutrition details for specific foods).

Remember that most of the fats in your diet will come from protein, but you can supplement with fattier foods like avocados, almonds, almond butter, and cooking oils like olive and coconut. Carbohydrates can primarily come from white rice, potatoes, and sweet potatoes. Why choose white rice over brown rice? The brown stuff contains substances that can prevent nutrients from being absorbed. "White rice has had the hull removed, leaving only the starch, which is all your body requires to replenish the glucose stores that power your training," explains Miyaki. Brown rice does contain more vitamins and minerals, but that is what vegetables are for. You can eat a lot of green vegetables; there is no limit on how much you should eat.

"After your weight workouts, you can have one slice of whole fruit," says Miyaki. "Fruit is a quick-digesting carbohydrate source that can provide your body with instant recovery fuel." It's a better option than carb powder, which, according to Miyaki, can spike your insulin and trigger rebound hypoglycemia—the crash after a sugary meal that can deplete your energy for hours. An apple or banana fits well, with a total carbohydrate content of around 30 grams.

Dairy, grains, and refined foods are all bad for your diet. Although they can provide valuable nutrients, most people have an allergy to them, causing digestive distress. If you don't mind eating dairy or grains in moderation, go ahead and do so, but you'll get quicker and better results if you stick to the foods on our list.

Training's Role

Working out does not burn enough calories to get rid of stubborn fat, but it does make you more muscular, which boosts your metabolism and helps you remain lean once you've reached your ideal weight. "Standard weight training is fine," Krahn says. "Do a heavy upper and lower body day, followed by two light days later in the week." Heavy days can restrict reps to 5–8, while lighter workouts can range from 8–15. "Alternatively, you could perform three full-body workouts a week." Since abs are primarily the product of proper nutrition, exercises that isolate them are not strictly necessary; however, one to three ab moves per session are permissible.

Cardio is not needed for fat loss. It is, however, necessary for optimum heart health and conditioning to engage in some type of cardiovascular exercise three to five days per week.

What's the Best Food to Eat After a Workout?

You already know that you should eat properly before working out, but post-exercise nutrition is also essential.

What you eat after a workout will help replenish your body and enhance recovery — and depending on the strength of your workout, if you skip a post-workout snack entirely, you might be losing out on a chance to boost protein synthesis, which is essential for muscle repair and development.

So, what are the best post-workout foods? These six-pointers will help you make the most of your post-workout window.

1. Consider the Intensity and Duration of Your Workout

What you eat — and when you eat it — depends on what you're doing and how long you're doing it.

"This decision will be focused on how fast you need to recover," says Michelle Duncan, R.D.N., a sports dietetics and nutrition specialist. "However, most people would be in good health to eat within an hour or two of most forms of exercise," she says.

However, if you are an elite athlete who does several workouts in a day, you may want to refuel immediately after a workout.

And, if you're doing an especially long or hard workout, Denise Reid, R.D. recommends eating within 30 minutes of your workout.

2. Combine Protein and Carbohydrates

Reid suggests aiming for 20 to 30 grams of high-quality protein and 30 to 40 grams of carbohydrates while preparing your post-workout meal.

Do you need inspiration? Here are a few safer alternatives:

- a protein-packed smoothie served with a turkey veggie sandwich wrap up
- a quinoa bowl topped with vegetables and chicken
- a peanut butter sandwich and a glass of chocolate milk

Duncan suggests tuna and crackers, a banana with peanut butter, or a protein shake for a lighter snack. "Protein shakes can be a simple way to satisfy your post-workout hydration and nutrition needs," Duncan says.

3. Do Not Skip Meals

"Skipping a meal and then waiting several hours to eat is the worst strategy," Michelle warns. "If you do that, you will not be able to restore glycogen to your muscles or obtain the required carbs and protein for recovery."

4. Avoid alcoholic beverages and high-fat foods.

You may have run a 5K where a post-race beer was part of the celebrations, but alcohol should not be part of your postworkout schedule in general, according to Michael, because it may hinder the training gains and recovery phase.

Snacks high in saturated fat and low in nutrient value can also be avoided. A snack with some healthy fats, such as avocado slices, is good after a workout, but anything too greasy can cause bloating.

5. Eat Healthily During the Day

Don't restrict your healthy eating habits to post-workout meals and snacks. Denise advises eating healthy meals and nutrient-dense snacks at regular intervals during the day.

If you're doing many workouts, she recommends increasing the carbohydrate intake during the day.

6. Always remember to hydrate.

Along with having the right nutrient blend, make sure you're staying hydrated, no matter what kind of workout you've done.

Also, low-impact or slower-paced workout sessions, such as a yoga class, should provide post-exercise rehydration.

You can find beverages developed explicitly at the supermarket to provide an optimum combination of carbohydrates, electrolytes, and water that will help you remain hydrated throughout your workout.

What's the bottom line? Consider post-workout eating to be an integral part of your overall fitness plan, rather than an afterthought, and it will help you achieve your goals faster.

6 Superfoods to Get a Beach Body

With the summer months almost here—many college students will graduate this Mother's Day, and your high schoolers will graduate soon—one thing is on everyone's mind: the beach! And, of course, how you'll appear on said sand.

Since we want you to feel confident and have the flat stomach you've been fantasizing about since, like, summer 2015, here's a list of superfoods that are rich in nutrients and, more importantly, endorse fat burning. If you pair a thoughtful diet with a fitness regiment (yeah, you'll have to do that as well), by August, when you hit the sands in your new suit and sunglasses, you'll have people looking up to you.

<u>1. Bananas</u>

The first point to remember is that sodium is extremely toxic. In all seriousness. Salt and salty foods (think chip snacks and anything highly processed) cause the body to hold water. And retaining a boatload of water causes you to swell and your tummy to appear bigger than it would otherwise.

Is there a solution? Aside from lowering your sodium intake, choose a potassium-rich snack, such as bananas. Potassium is a super nutrient because it flushes out excess water and salt from your body, leaving you looking lean.

2. Sweet Potatoes

Not all potatoes are the same! We're not just talking about french fries here. Regular potatoes have a higher GI rating than sweet potatoes, and the higher the GI rating, the more likely the carbohydrate content of a food is to affect your blood sugar.

This is not just a problem for diabetics. Foods with lower GI values (around 55 or lower) digest more slowly, reducing insulin resistance and aiding in the prevention of calorie conversion to fat. When sweet potatoes are boiled (rather than baked, for example), they have a low GI score in the 40s. Furthermore, sweet potatoes are high in vitamins such as B6, C, and A.

3. Nuts

Snacks are permissible on occasion. Instead of flaming hot Cheetos, try some nuts!

Nuts provide good fat (yes, such a thing exists) that can nourish your body while also turning off fat genes. The highfat content of nuts (walnuts, almonds, etc.) will also help keep you from feeling hungry in between meals, preventing you from making a pit stop at Carl's Jr. for some giant burger that will leave you depressed and feeling like a fat ass five minutes after consumption.

By the way, peanuts are technically a legume. So, stick to natural nuts that are finely salted or unsalted

4. Green tea

Okay, maybe you don't eat it, but the catechins in green tea are antioxidants that cause fat cells to release fat. It also explicitly targets your tum tum. It also stimulates the liver to burn the fat and use it as energy after being released. In other words, if you don't like hot tea, you'd better start soon if you want to look nice in your suit and shades.

5. Salmon

It is important to consume lean protein. If you want to grow a more toned (or even ripped!) body, you must feed your hungry muscles after your workout. Salmon is lean meat high in protein and omega-3s, all of which help reduce fat accumulation and combat inflammation.

6. Apples

Apples are awesome. They're delicious, but they're also low in calories and a good source of fiber. In addition, fiber helps reduce fat and encourage weight loss, even in the absence of a comprehensive diet plan.

Tips to Get Beach Body Quickly

Summer can't come fast enough! All of the months spent indoors waiting for warm weather will be rewarded when you put on your bathing suit. If the idea of wearing a pair of swim shorts makes you nervous, there is still time to prepare!

Don't worry, we're not talking about dangerous, extreme diets that deprive you of food and leave you exhausted or irritated. Instead, we've created this beach body guide that everyone can use to get a body they'll be proud of!

1. <u>Consume protein at any meal.</u>

It goes without saying that getting enough protein is vital for increasing muscle mass, but protein also helps with fat loss. According to a report published in the American Journal of Clinical Nutrition, spreading your protein consumption through all three meals will help you lose weight. After analyzing 24 studies on protein intake, the researchers discovered that people who ate protein during the day lost more weight while retaining more lean mass - the ultimate target for the perfect beach body.

2. <u>Quit snacking.</u>

Snacking, even healthy snacking, will cause weight loss to stall and keep you from losing those last few pounds.

A few fast bites of healthy food may not seem to be much, but the hurried and sometimes mindless way most people snack can be detrimental to getting beach body ready. A few extra calories here and there add up easily and can lead to accidental overeating. Instead of snacking, eat three to four nutritious meals a day. When you have set meal times, it is much easier to keep track of your intake.

3. <u>Avoid alcoholic beverages such as cocktails, wine, and beer.</u>

Is your ideal beach body leaner and more toned than your present physique? Then you must reduce your calorie intake so that your body can start burning stored fat. You are consuming needless calories with each drink of alcohol. In reality, according to a study published in the American Journal of Clinical Nutrition, men eat an additional 433 calories on days when they only have a couple of drinks. Furthermore, alcohol lowers our inhibitions and makes us less likely to adhere to our diets. If you want to keep your beach body slim, stay away from the bar.

5. Eat a low-bloat diet.

Your beach body will appear puffy rather than shredded if you have a bloated stomach. If you only have a few days before your beach body reveals, stick to a low-bloat diet. To begin, avoid high-sodium packaged foods, which can cause water retention. Surprisingly, some nutritious foods may also induce bloating. Broccoli and kale are examples of cruciferous vegetables that contain slow-digesting carbohydrates that can trigger gas. Apples, beans, and peas are several other healthy foods that can induce bloating. Eat potassium-rich fruits like bananas, avocados, kiwis, and oranges to avoid water retention. Asparagus and cucumbers are the best vegetables for bloating. Don't be alarmed if you get bloated. To cure the condition, try this all-natural homemade tonic.

6. Get 8 hours of sleep each night.

Sleep is important for achieving any physical goals. If your ideal beach body calls for significant fat loss or big muscle gain, sleep will be critical to your success. Sleep enables the body to heal from strenuous exercise, as well as develop and strengthen muscles. Sleep deprivation will disturb your hormonal balance, leading to excessive hunger and cravings.

Sleep deprivation will weaken your willpower, causing you to miss workouts and cheat on your diet.

According to the American Journal of Clinical Nutrition, sleep-deprived people snack later at night and are more likely to prefer high-carb snacks.

7. Do not overlook the upper back exercise.

A beach body isn't full unless it has a slender waist. Most people are unaware that strong, well-developed upper back muscles make the waist appear smaller and more formed. When you fail to exercise your upper back, your body will appear out of shape, and your waist will appear larger than it is. Begin sculpting the upper back that your beach body needs by incorporating bent-over rows into your workout routine.

Dumbbell Rows with a Bent Over Position

- Hold a dumbbell in each hand with your palms facing each other.
- Bring your body forward by bending at the hip and bending your knees slightly. Maintain a straight spine and a chest that is almost parallel to the floor.
- Allow the dumbbells to hang in front of you so that your arms are perpendicular to the floor.

- Exhale as you lift the dumbbells to your sides, keeping your elbows close to your body and your torso stationary.
- Squeeze the shoulder blades together and stay for a second at the end of the movement.
- Inhale as you gradually lower the dumbbells back to their starting spot. Repeat for the recommended number of times.

8. Work on your stance.

It's difficult to flaunt an amazing beach body if the posture is abysmal. Poor posture is not only unsightly, but it can also impede preparation. Bad posture can trigger a cascade of structural defects that result in acute issues, such as joint pain throughout your body, decreased flexibility, and weakened muscles, all of which can impair your ability to burn fat and create strength." Almost everybody will benefit from the better posture.

9. To lose weight, use high-intensity interval training.

High-intensity interval training (HIIT) is a form of conditioning workout in which short bursts of recovery follow short bursts of high-intensity exercise. When opposed to conventional cardio, HIIT is a much more time-efficient method of fat loss. For example, researchers at the University of Western Ontario discovered that making 4 to 6 30-second sprints (with 4-minute rests in between) burned more fat than slogging through 60 minutes of incline treadmill walking.

10. Boost your non-exercise physical activity.

Maintaining a healthy diet and exercise regimen will go a long way toward making you look good on the beach. However, you can also consider what you do outside of the gym and the kitchen. Increasing your non-exercise physical activity will improve your training outcomes and make it easier to keep your beach body long into the fall. Simple improvements such as using the stairs instead of the elevator, walking for relaxation instead of channel surfing, and being involved on weekends will make a huge difference.

11. Choose exercises that focus on the heart.

Everyone's beach body checklist includes a solid, firm heart. Pick exercises that require extra core strength to incorporate extra core training into your workout. Choose pushups instead of bench press, front squats and deadlifts instead of cable rows, and bodyweight rows instead of cable rows.

Weighted hip thrusts will help you shape your glutes.

Every pair of swim trunks looks great with a good collection of glutes! In order to achieve a wellrounded beach body, incorporate hip thrusts into your workout.

Hip thrust

- Sit on the floor with your back against one side of a bench or box, shoulder blades resting on the edge, arms at your sides, and knees bent to a 90-degree angle.
- Exhale, force your feet into the dirt and lift your hips up to build a straight line from your knees to your shoulders by squeezing your glutes as tightly as possible. Take care

not to arch your lower back into hyperextension. Throughout the exercise, keep the ribcage and pelvis tucked against each other.
- Inhale, drop your hips to the floor while raising your upper body, and return to the starting spot.
- Tip: You can make this exercise more difficult by crossing your hips with an Olympic bar loaded with weights.

It's finally time to get started. The beach body of your dreams is closer than you thought. Consider how much more selfassurance you would have in a matter of weeks. Furthermore, you achieved your target without subjecting your body to an unhealthy crash diet.

Following this beach body guide for a smarter fitness schedule, high-quality nutrition strategy, and re-energizing sleep will help you achieve the body you want in much less time than you thought possible.

Top 6 Foods to Avoid for a Beach Body

Is summer on the horizon? Do you want to look nice for a class reunion or a family reunion? If your body isn't quite where you want it to be, it may be time to reconsider your diet.

Whatever is triggering your love-hate relationship with your swim trunks, whether it's a few extra pounds or too much bloating in the midsection, the reality is that it's most likely your diet to blame. "You are what you eat" is true—if you eat fattening, non-nutritious foods all the time, you will not feel safe or confident.

If you want to improve your diet and see real results, here are six foods to avoid (most of the time):

1. Oil-fried foods

What are the similarities between wings, doughnuts, fried chicken, and French fries? (Aside from the fact that it tastes great?) They're all good friends in the oil industry. This gives them that crispy texture, but it also adds a lot of calories and fat. This is due to the fact that up to 25% of the oil used in frying is consumed by the food. Depending on the food, this may cause a significant increase in fat and calorie intake. A boneless, skinless chicken breast, for example, has 124 calories, but a battered and fried chicken breast has 294 calories—more than double!

If you want to lose weight and show off your muscles at the beach, avoid fried foods in favor of baked or grilled alternatives. Ignore something on the menu that says "super crispy"; that's code for "deep-friend."

2. Processed junk foods

You know the ones: chips, cookies, and donuts. Although these foods can taste good, they are the epitome of "empty calories": foods with no nutritional value that leave you hungry and unsatisfied. It's a never-ending loop.

This form of junk food contains a lot of processed sugar. Too much added sugar in the diet (more than 10% of total calories, according to new USDA guidelines) can cause a slew of health issues, including an increased risk of heart disease and, finally, type 2 diabetes.

If you're hungry, satisfy your hunger with swimsuit-friendly snacks like nuts, Greek yogurt, or berries.

3. Sugary drinks and alcoholic beverages

Soda, lemonade, frozen coffees, and adult beverages are summer staples, particularly for warm-weather gatherings and weekend brunch on the patio (mimosas, anyone?). However, these beverages are often high in sugar. To give you an example, an iced caramel latte has the same amount of sugar as three donuts—nearly 9 teaspoons in just one drink!

Sugary drinks will not help you lose weight if you're trying to fit into your swimsuit. Numerous studies have linked this liquid candy to an increased risk of obesity and type 2 diabetes.

The USDA issued updated dietary recommendations in 2015, recommending that added sugar consumption be limited to less than 10% of total calories. That is just 180 calories for a 1,800 calorie diet (or 45g sugar). Given that one daily can of soda contains 39 g of sugar, it's easy to see how sugary beverages can easily add up.

Going out for drinks with your friends? By using club soda mixers and water, you can avoid sugary liquids. If the idea of drinking water bores you, ask the bartender to add lemon/lime wedges, mint leaves, and/or a splash of cranberry or grapefruit juice. Alternatively, allow yourself one cocktail of your choice before switching to the club soda mixer.

4. Fatty meat cuts

For you meat-eaters, the hot dogs, burgers, and brats that most of us enjoy at summer barbecues practically clog the arteries with saturated fats, AGEs, and a lot of calories—the last thing you want when you're trying to get swimsuit ready.

A diet high in saturated fat can also shorten your life. Red meat intake has been related to an increased risk of cardiovascular disease and other health issues in study after study. One study discovered a link between processed red meat and death; only one extra serving of processed red meat per day increased the risk of death by 20%.

While the occasional juicy burger is perfect, make sure your protein comes from lean sources such as chicken breasts, fish, or even plant-based protein powders.

5. White flour

White flour has a poor reputation. To be frank, it is welldeserved. It not only lacks nutritional value, but it is frequently high in carbohydrates and sugar while being low in protein—the ideal formula for an insulin spike and sugar drop.

Some of the worst offenders are pasta, bagels, pizza crust, pastries, cakes, and cookies. They're also high in calories, which isn't synonymous with having a "beach body." Fortunately, there are healthier options that are nevertheless delicious. Try making pasta out of quinoa or lentils. If you're craving Italian, try new healthier choices like spaghetti squash. When it comes to baking, whole grain and multigrain bread are much superior to white-flour bread.

6. Pizza
==

Pizza, no matter how balanced we try to make it by sprinkling a few veggies on top, isn't doing your body any favors. The majority of store-bought or delivered pizzas have a lot of cheese and meat on top of a thick, white bread dough. Basically, everything we just said was detrimental to your health. Not only that, but it's difficult to stop at only one slice of pizza when it comes to portion control.

If you're craving pizza but don't want to jeopardize your search for the ideal beach body, try cooking it at home. You'll probably use healthy ingredients and have better portion control. Cauliflower crust can be used to make a truly nutritious pizza. When you do order pizza, go for a thin crust with veggie toppings.

In conclusion
==

Don't stress if your summer body isn't exactly where you want it to be. It isn't too late! Avoiding these swimsuitsabotaging foods will assist you in losing weight. And if you do make a mistake and overindulge, don't be too hard on yourself. Simply get back on track and select healthy foods the next time.

How to prevent bloating after a meal

Bloating after eating is normally not a cause for concern, and it is also avoidable by adopting certain simple habits such as eating less fiber, avoiding carbonated beverages, and eating and drinking more slowly.

Being bloated after a meal is a common occurrence for most people. It may make the stomach swell and feel bloated, and it may be followed by flatulence or burping.

Although bloating after eating is not uncommon, there are a few things you can do to prevent it. In this post, we'll look at ten ways to avoid bloating.

Ten ways to stop post-meal bloating

The following suggestions can help minimize or avoid postmeal bloating:

1. Limit your fiber intake.

Fiber is a type of carbohydrate found in plant-based foods that the body is unable to digest. It serves many important roles in the body, including aiding in blood sugar levels and sugar intake regulation.

High-fiber foods, on the other hand, may cause excessive gas production in some people. According to one studyTrusted Source, a low-fiber diet helped alleviate bloating in people with idiopathic constipation.

High-fiber foods contain the following:

- legumes
- fruits, like oranges and apples
- oats, whole grain
- peas that have been split
- broccoli

- Brussels sprouts

2. Be mindful of food allergies and intolerances.

Bloating is a common sign of food intolerance or allergy. Excessive gas output or gas trapped in the gastrointestinal tract may be caused by intolerances and allergies. Wheat and gluten are the most likely culprits.

Since there are no accurate ways to detect a particular food disorder or allergy, the only way to identify them is by trial and error. Keeping a food diary will help you monitor which foods are causing symptoms like bloating.

3. Limit the intake of high-fat foods.

Fat is a valuable source of energy and is an integral component of every healthy diet. Fats are digested slowly by the body because they take longer than most other foods to pass through the digestive tract and can cause stomach emptying to be delayed. Bloating can occur in some people as a result of this.

People who experience this can find that avoiding high-fat foods helps to minimize bloating. Research of people with stomach-emptying disorders, for example, discovered that high-fat solid meals increased symptoms such as bloating.

4. Slowly drinking and eating

Drinking or eating too quickly increases the amount of air a person swallows, which can cause more gas to accumulate in the gastrointestinal tract.

Bloating can be caused by people who eat or drink quickly; slowing down the rate at which they eat can help to alleviate the problem.

5. Avoid carbonated beverages.

Carbonated beverages contain carbon dioxide, a gas that can accumulate in the digestive tract and cause bloating. Diet forms of fizzy drinks may also cause this.

Still, water is the perfect alternative to carbonated beverages for reducing bloating.

6. Ginger

Ginger has long been used as a digestive aid. It contains carminative, which aids in the reduction of excess gas in the gastrointestinal tract.

According to a 2013 report, ginger has several health benefits, including the relief of gastrointestinal problems such as bloating.

7. Avoid using chewing gum.

When an individual chews gum, he or she swallows more air. In certain people, this air can accumulate in the gastrointestinal tract and cause bloating.

8. Do some light exercise after eating.

Some people can benefit from light exercise after eating, such as going for a walk. According to research, moderate physical activity helps expel gas from the gastrointestinal tract and relieves bloating.

9. Try not to talk while feeding.

Speaking when feeding increases the likelihood of swallowing air. This may result in an accumulation of air in the gastrointestinal tract, resulting in bloating.

10. Treatment of heartburn

Heartburn happens as stomach acid flows back up the throat, causing an unpleasant burning feeling. Bloating is also a common symptom of it.

For certain individuals, treating heartburn may be an effective way of minimizing bloating. Over-the-counter drugs such as antacids may be used to treat heartburn.

What triggers post-meal bloating?

Bloating happens in the abdomen. It occurs when a significant volume of air or gas accumulates in the gastrointestinal tract.

Eating is a common cause of bloating because the body releases gas as it digests food. When people eat or drink, they also swallow air, which enters the gastrointestinal tract. Flatulence and burping normally help to reduce gas and air buildup in the stomach.

Bloating is a symptom of many of medical conditions, including irritable bowel syndrome and food intolerance.
Most instances of bloating, however, are avoidable.

OBSTACLE IN OUR PATH

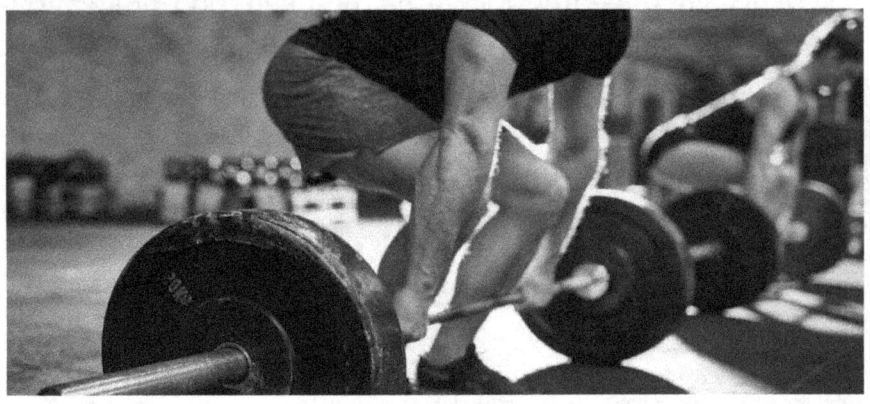

It's hard enough to get in shape, however, there are additional difficulties that accompany attempting to get fit. Here are some common difficulties individuals face when getting fit.

6 Common Issues When Getting Fit

1. Not Keeping A Proper Sleep Schedule

Chemicals assume a significant part in keeping up fat and muscle. Not getting sufficient rest by keeping awake until late or keeping an ill-advised rest timetable will effectively disturb your circadian musicality and result in not gathering muscle building or weight reduction objectives. Hitting the hay early and getting up early is the ideal rest plan for your chemicals. The sun's enactment of our pineal organ and its relationship with attentiveness is so significant.

2. Thinking Things Will Change Overnight

It might take a few months or more to accomplish the physical body make-up you're searching for. Crash diets and starving yourself won't work over the long haul, so you need to acknowledge you're in it for the long stretch. Stay away from crash counts calories, and don't starve yourself. Attempt and not spotlight on your eating regimen or practice and simply fuse it into your life and go on with your day. Wellness applications can help extensively in such a manner. You can set the wellness application to help you remember your eating regimen and wellness objectives and approach your life.

3. Practicing Too Much

Over-practicing will simply exhaustion you and channel your chemical levels. Focus on an activity schedule that actuates your muscles yet doesn't continue for quite a long time. Serious, enduring activity will, in general, leave you needing simple calories. Extreme focus irregular cardio is an extraordinary technique to lean out your physical make-up without exhaustion. Once more, utilizing a wellness application is an excellent method to monitor your activity, so you don't try too hard.

4. Being Nervous At The Gym

The rec center resembles some other public spot. Individuals stay out of other people's affairs, and you don't really need to converse with any other individual. That being said, on the off chance that you feel threatened, you can generally attempt another rec center. Another option is to wear your earphones and spotlight the music. The weight lifting territory can be particularly scary. It might take some time before you assemble up the fortitude to begin utilizing the loads and machines. It might appear to be an extraordinary region; however it's not, you can simply begin utilizing them like any other individual. For best outcomes, ask a mentor at your exercise center to show you around the loads territory and show you how to utilize anything you're new to.

5. Purchasing A Bunch of Supplements

Try not to squander your cash by purchasing a lot of enhancements. In the event that you have an absence of a couple of components in your body, it's OK to enhance as long as your primary care physician supports it. In any case, spending your cash on a ton of enhancements will sap your financial plan for more important things for your wellness, similar to quality food, exercise, and wellness applications. All things being equal, center around putting resources into the correct enhancements, and stay away from the ones that aren't powerful, saving you both exertion and time.

6. Stress

Stress, despondency, or anything that is taking up a ton of your passionate energy will effectively destroy any weight reduction or wellness objectives you have. Your adrenal organs will get exhausted, and you will get yourself incapable of summoning the energy for your day-by-day practice schedule. Attempt and discover what's disturbing you and take out the wellspring of stress. This is a principal reason many individuals experience difficulty with getting fit.

Negative Mind Patterns When Getting Fit

Many questions arise while getting exercise. Some persons show excuses, someone gets de-motivated, and some get disappointed. After all, Adhering to a standard exercise plan isn't simple. All things considered, there are a lot of possible impediments — time, fatigue, wounds, fearlessness. However, these issues don't have to hinder you. Think about viable methodologies for conquering regular boundaries to wellness.

1. I need more an ideal opportunity to work out

Putting to the side opportunity to exercise can be a test. Utilize a little inventiveness to take advantage of your time. Press in short strolls for the day. On the off chance that you don't possess energy for a full exercise, don't stress over it. Any measure of action is superior to none by any means. More limited eruptions of activity, for example, going for short stroll breaks a couple of times during the day, offer advantages as well. Intend to move gradually up to practicing around 30 minutes on most days of the week.

Rise prior. In the event that your days are stuffed and the evening hours are occupied, get up 30 minutes sooner a couple of times each week to work out. Whenever you've changed in accordance with early-morning exercises, add one more little while to the daily practice.

Drive less, walk more. Park in the back column of the parking garage or even a couple of squares away and stroll to your objective.

Redo your ceremonies. Your week after week Saturday early showing with the children or your closest companion could be reawakened as your week after week Saturday bicycle ride, rock-climbing exercise or excursion to the pool.

2. I think practice is exhausting

It's regular to become tired of a dreary exercise for quite a while, particularly when you're going it single-handedly. However, practice doesn't need to be exhausting.

Pick exercises you appreciate. You'll be bound to remain intrigued. Keep in mind, whatever makes you move checks.

Differ the daily schedule. Turn among a few exercises — like strolling, swimming and cycling — to cause you to remain alert while molding distinctive muscle gatherings.

Unite. Exercise with companions, family members, neighbors or collaborators. You'll appreciate the fellowship and the gathering's support.

Investigate new choices. Master new abilities while getting in an exercise. Look at practice classes or sports associations at an entertainment place or fitness center.

3. I'm hesitant about what I look like

Try not to get down on yourself! Advise yourself that you're improving your cardiovascular wellbeing or spotlight on how much more grounded you feel after an exercise.

Keep away from the group. In case you're awkward practicing around others, go solo from the start. Attempt an activity video or a movement situated computer game. Or then again, think about putting resources into a fixed bike, treadmill, step climbing machine or another piece of home gym equipment.

Zero in on what's to come. Recognition yourself for making a guarantee to your wellbeing. What's more, recollect that as you become fitter and more open to working out, your selfassurance is probably going to improve too.

4. I'm too worn out to even consider practicing after work

No energy to work out? Without work out, you'll have no energy. It's a cycle. Yet, breaking the cycle with actual work is probably the best blessing you can give yourself. Also, over the long haul, exercise can help improve your rest quality and your energy level.

Attempt a morning portion of activity. Recollect the idea to get up 30 minutes sooner to work out? Jump on the treadmill or fixed bike while you tune in to the radio or watch the morning news. Or, on the other hand, venture outside for a lively walk.

Make the most of noon. Keep a couple of strolling shoes at your work area, and go for an energetic stroll during your mid-day break.

Be readied. Ensure you have agreeable shoes and loosefitting garments for working out. Take them with you to the shopping center or when you travel.

5. I'm too languid to even consider working out

On the off chance that the prospect of a morning run makes you tired, think about a few plans to get rolling.

Set reasonable assumptions. On the off chance that you set your objectives excessively high, you may surrender easily. Start with a stroll around the square. Try not to surrender in the event that you get a handle on worn. Go for another stroll around the square tomorrow. Keep it up, and ultimately you'll presently don't understand worn.

Work with your temperament, not against it. Plan active work for times when you will, in general, feel fierier or possibly not exactly so sluggish.

Timetable exercise as you would plan a significant arrangement. Square off occasions in your schedule for active work, and ensure your loved ones know about your responsibility. Request their consolation and backing.

6. I'm not athletic

You needn't bother with the common athletic capacity to be dynamic. Regardless of whether you've been idle for quite a while, it's not very late to get more dynamic.

Keep it straightforward. Have a go at something essential, like an everyday walk. Start gradually and allow your body to become acclimated to the expanded action.

Discover organization. Pick an action you like, like moving or planting, and welcome companions to participate. You'll have some good times while helping each other work out.

Disregard the opposition. Try not to stress overturning into a genius competitor or joining the hard-bodied competitors at the wellness club. Essentially center around the positive changes you're making to your body and brain.

7. I've attempted to practice previously and fizzled

Try not to surrender. Reexamine what turned out badly and gain from your errors. In spite of the fact that you can't generally see apparent changes when you bring down your danger of diabetes, hypertension or coronary illness, you can have a beneficial outcome in your wellbeing through regular exercise.

Speed yourself. Start little and develop to more serious exercises later, when your body is prepared.

Set reasonable objectives. Try not to guarantee yourself you will turn out for an hour consistently and get down on yourself when you miss the mark. Stick with sensible objectives you can accomplish, for example, practicing 20 minutes per day, three days per week for the main month.

Recollect why you're working out. Utilize your own wellness objectives as inspiration, and prize yourself as you meet your objectives.

8. I can't manage the cost of gym charges

You needn't bother with a rec center enrollment to get an extraordinary exercise. Think about rational other options.

Do fortifying activities at home. Utilize cheap obstruction groups — lengths of versatile tubing that come in differing qualities — instead of loads. Do pushups or squats utilizing your body weight.

Start a mobile gathering. Gather together companions, neighbors or colleagues for normal gathering strolls. Plan courses through your area or close to your work environment, along with neighborhood stops and trails, or in a close-by shopping center.

Use the stairwell. Avoid the lift when you can. Even better, make climbing steps an exercise in itself.

Attempt your public venue. Exercise classes offered through a neighborhood entertainment division or local area training gathering may better accommodate your financial plan than a yearly rec center enrollment.

9. I'm apprehensive I'll harm myself on the off chance that I work out

In case you're apprehensive about harming yourself, get going with basic exercises, for example, strolling and take it gradually.

Take it gradually. Start with a straightforward strolling program. Warm-up before you exercise, and cool down when you're done. As you become more sure about your capacities, add new exercises to your daily schedule.

Attempt an activity class for amateurs. You'll take in the fundamentals by beginning all along.

Get professional assistance. Get a wellness instructional exercise from a guaranteed master who can screen your developments and point you the correct way. On the off chance that you've had a past injury or you have an ailment, you might need to counsel your primary care physician or an activity specialist for help planning a workout schedule fitting for you.

10. My family doesn't uphold my endeavors

Help those near you remember the advantages of standard exercise and bring them along to work out.

Kick-off your children. Pursue a parent-youngster practice class. Pack an excursion lunch and take your family to the recreation center for a round of tag or kickball. Sprinkle with the children in the pool as opposed to watching from your seat.

Propose another experience. Rather than recommending an exercise at the rec center, welcome a companion to go to an indoor climbing divider or lease a two-person bike for the end of the week.

Perform twofold responsibility. Volunteer to drive your youngsters to the shopping center, and afterward, walk laps inside while you hang tight for the customers. What's more, take a stab at strolling around your youngster's school during exercises, practices or practices.

In the event that essential, show at least a bit of kindness toheart talk with your friends and family. On the off chance that they don't share your wellness aspirations, ask them to in any event, regard your craving to get fit.

Since you know you're in good company to manage these wellness challenges, it very well may be simpler to deal with every one of them. Keep in mind, wellness is a way of life, not a momentary venture. When you get fit as a fiddle, it will be simpler to confront every one of the difficulties referenced previously.

MOTIVATIONAL QUOTES TO INSPIRE YOU TOWARD YOUR GOAL

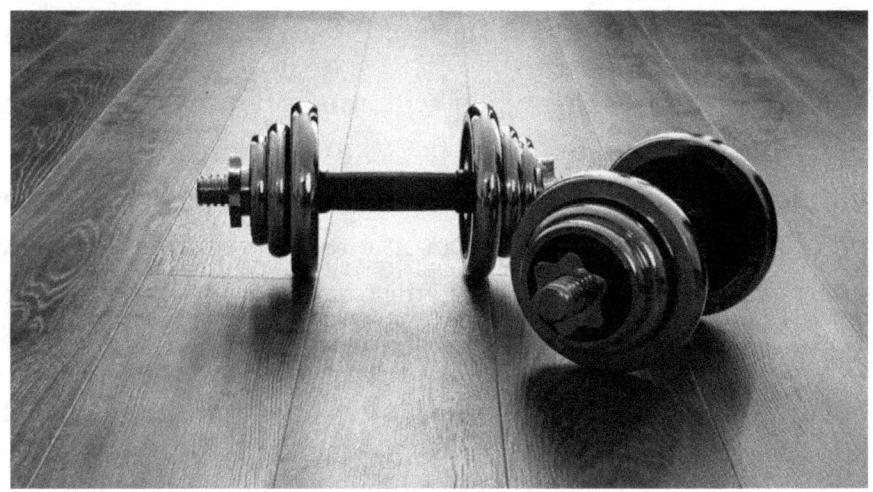

This 4 weeks program may look too hard. 28 days of hard work to get that beach body you always dreamed of.

The 28 inspiring fitness quotes below will motivate you to get started on your new workout routine and get your exercise game on.

Having our own dream image of our best summer body is enough inspiration to begin working out for some of us. Who doesn't want to look and feel great in their favorite bathing suit? Putting forth the effort to make the vision a reality, on the other hand, does not come as easily to others. When exercise isn't in your blood, squeezing your body into swimwear might not be as appealing.

Fitness isn't just about appearances, and exercise is beneficial to your wellbeing whether or not you care about losing even an ounce of weight. And, regardless of who you are or what fitness goals you wish to achieve, we all know that the most difficult part of achieving something is always having the first burst of strength to get up and get started.

This is particularly true when beginning a new exercise regimen. You must acclimate your body to working out again or differently, which is seldom enjoyable. You'll be achy. It can be painful at times. It can also become tedious at times. However, once you get into a routine, exercise can become the best kind of everyday habit.

Finally, when you get into the habit of working out, you feel fantastic. When you feel healthy on the inside, and out, it makes it better in the end.

Here are my choices for the top 28 best health and workout inspiration quotes to get you out there and exercise!

1. Once you start, you won't want to stop.
2. Don't forget why you started.
3. Don't quit.
4. Convince your mind.
5. Don't discourage yourself.
6. Everyone goes at their own pace.
7. Keep your mentality strong.
8. Don't get in your way.
9. Work for what you want.

10. No excuses.
11. Think about the results.
12. The pain is a good sign.
13. The hardest things are worth it.
14. Get serious.
15. You will see the results of your hard work.
16. Never give up!
17. Think a positive way.
18. Embrace the pain.
19. Perseverance is key.
20. Look amazing.
21. Baby steps can help.
22. Heading in the right direction.
23. Just go workout.
24. It's all about loving yourself.
25. Don't let slow progress discourage you.
26. Show it off.
27. This is true.
28. It all comes down to you.

CPSIA information can be obtained
at www.ICGtesting.com
Printed in the USA
LVHW021726090521
686930LV00013B/781